MW01715021

Creative Calories & Recipes for Weight Gain

Featuring Distinguished Chefs

Debbie Kaufman
LaurieAnn Scher, MS, RD, CDE
Melanie Katrinak, RD, CSP, LDN

Craving Calories, is a registered trademark. All other trademarks referenced within this publication are the property of their respective owners. Craving Calories LLC, is not affiliated with or endorsed by any manufacturer, product, restaurant or chef within this publication.

The views and information expressed in this publication are those of the authors and are not meant to dictate, guide, or provide medical treatment. Each patient is unique and should be individually evaluated and treated. The authors disclaim responsibility for the application of the information contained herein.

Every attempt has been made to ensure that the information presented in this book is correct, but there remains the possibility of error for which the authors cannot be held responsible. The information provided was verified at the time of the publication, but, manufacturers may change ingredients, formulations or processes in manufacturing their products that would affect their calorie content and compositions. We advise you to verify the content and composition with the manufacturer before purchasing a product. This information is not intended as and does not substitute for medical advice – the information presented is for patient education only. Please see your personal physician for further evaluation of your individual case.

No book, including this one, can replace the services of a qualified health professional.

The views and opinions expressed by the authors are their own and do not reflect those of their employers.

*Anyone experiencing Dysphagia or an eating disorder should consult with their medical treatment team regarding appropriate use of this book.

Copyright © 2013 by:
Debbie Kaufman
LaurieAnn Scher, MS,RD, CDE
Melanie Katrinak, RD, CSP, LDN

All rights reserved.
ISBN: 0615889697
ISBN-13: 978-0615889696

Forward/Dedication

Creative Calories & Recipes for Weight Gain is a cookbook created to help the millions of people who are struggling to maintain or gain weight due to various medical conditions, genetics or other reasons. Weight loss might result in people suffering from conditions such as Cancer, Aging, Depression, ADD/ADHD, OCD, Growth Hormone Deficiency and Cystic Fibrosis, to name a few. While suffering with our daughter through major weight loss, I was surprised by the lack of resources available to help her gain weight. I have spent many years trying my best to meet the challenge of adding calories to meals wherever possible, while constantly trying to keep a new twist on these preparations. This is my dream: the creation of a cookbook and resource to aid all those who may encounter weight loss and help them so they do not go through this alone. This cookbook contains over 100 delicious recipes from distinguished chefs of leading restaurants across the United States and recipe favorites from family and friends. In addition to recipes, it offers helpful and invaluable information related to appetite, eating and weight gain.

This cookbook is dedicated to our beautiful daughter Lea, who has a wonderful spirit, smile, and love of life. When our daughter was 12, many events had taken place which triggered a fear of choking and she became afraid to eat or swallow, causing hospitalization and a true medical concern.

Through this experience and meeting people with other conditions, I realized that there is a huge population of both children and adults for whom calorie intake is critical. While many cookbooks are trying to help others lose weight, there are a large number of people who need to learn how to maximize caloric intake to maintain or gain weight. The **Creative Calories & Recipes for Weight Gain** cookbook includes a wide variety of recipes and calorie rich drink options along with information on weight gain, convenient calories to keep on hand, calorie boosting tips, metabolism, and calorie expenditure and compensation.

Many thanks to the Co-Authors of the **Creative Calories & Recipes for Weight Gain** cookbook: LaurieAnn Scher who worked tirelessly on this cookbook and Melanie Katrinak whose collaboration began years ago as an integral part of Lea's nutritional care team at The Children's Hospital of Philadelphia. Thank you to the incredible chefs, friends and family members who provided their time and recipes to help create this book.

Thank you to Dr. Donald Schwartz (current Health Commissioner of Philadelphia), and the entire dedicated Medical Team of The Children's Hospital of Philadelphia. Thank you to Lori Kasmen from the AAC in Bala Cynwyd, PA and her team, for their knowledge and dedication and thank you to Dr. Kathleen Schramm from SPA in Southampton, PA for her recommendations and guidelines.

Additionally, we are grateful to Dr. Jonathon Grayson from the AOTCP for his support, guidance and expertise, Dr. Martin Friedman from the University of Pennsylvania and all the others who have helped along the way: we thank you.

Special thanks to my inspirational and incredible husband who had the vision for this idea and our terrific son who came up with the name Craving Calories. Thank you to my cousin Stacy Kamisar, who graciously introduced me to LaurieAnn Scher, one of our co-authors and to Jon Kamisar for all his time and assistance with Craving Calories, LLC.

I could not have taken on this project without the help from all of the above.

Thank You!

To Continued Good Health!

Debbie

I would like to thank my husband Peter Goldman and my two sons, Zachary and Schuyler Goldmanscher who gave me the time and space to work on this book. Thank you to my mom, Evelyn Scher for providing her simple high calorie recipes for this book and thanks to her and my dad, Robert Scher for giving me the confidence to think that I could actually write a book. Thanks also to my sister, Julie Molinare who has not only been an inspiration, but a great resource answering my inane questions on websites and social marketing. Thanks to my brother, Daniel Scher for all his hard work from day one because he believed in me and the project. Thank you, thank you, thank you to Debbie Kaufman and Melanie Katrinak for more than anyone can ever imagine and finally, thanks to all of my wonderful patients who have taught me about food, eating, weight gain (and loss) and the human spirit.

Life, like food is better when it can be enjoyed,

laurieAnn

I would like to thank Lea Kaufman who became my inspiration to better understand and advocate for the unique and individual needs of each of my patients. A special thank you to Debbie Kaufman for choosing me to be part of this amazing project and giving me the opportunity to make such a contribution to society. Thank you to LaurieAnn Scher for sharing her time, expertise, support, and wisdom (both professional and personal) throughout this project. Thank you to Dr. Donald Schwartz and Dr. Kenneth Ginsburg for their understanding and support while working on their team. Thank you to Lori Enriquez and Rebecca Rogers for their encouragement, support and advice. Thank you to Carol Day for her recipe contributions and endless support and encouragement. A special thank you to Bill for his support and advice during this project. Thank you to Dr. Joel Pevar who was a healer and always encouraged and inspired me to help others and make such contributions to society.

Melanie

“One cannot think well, love well, sleep well, if one has not dined well. – Virginia Woolf

Table of Contents

Introduction Page 1

Chapter 1: First things First about Weight Gain Page 3

Remember Your Heart 5
Weight Gain in Children 6
Lighting and Atmosphere: How it Affects Appetite 8

Chapter 2: Metabolism and Exercise Page 9

Calorie Compensation 10

Chapter 3: Convenient Calories and Calorie Boosters Page 12

Foods to Keep on Hand to Add Calories & Nutrients 12

Chapter 4: Fast and Furious Calories Page 13

Fast Food Items with 700+ Calories by Restaurant 13
Fast Food Drinks/Shakes with 700+ Calories by Restaurant 15

Chapter 5: Distinguished Calories from Distinguished Chefs Page 17

Arpeggio. Springhouse, Pennsylvania Page 18

Mediterranean Mini Crust-less Quiche 18
Chocolate Bread Pudding Topped with Caramelized Bananas 19
Medjool Dates Stuffed with Mascarpone Cheese and Walnuts 21

Bayona. New Orleans, Louisiana Page 22

Smoked Duck Hash with Calvados Sauce 23

California School of Culinary Art. Los Angeles, California Page 25

JB's Cajun Potato Salad 25

Carlos Restaurant. Highland Park, Illinois Page 26

Mushroom Crusted Petit Filet Mignon with Butter Poached Fingerling Potatoes, Broccoli Raab and a Cabernet-Mushroom Reduction 27

Charlie Trotters. Chicago, Illinois **Page 29**

Goat Cheese and Basil Ravioli with Tomato Water 30

Rack of Lamb with Crispy Polenta and Mustard Sauce 32

Michel Richard Citronelle. Washington, DC **Page 34**

Chocolate Bar 35

Dante & Luigi's Corona di ferro. Philadelphia, Pennsylvania **Page 38**

Homemade Manicotti 39

Hudson's on the Bend. Austin, Texas **Page 40**

Appetizers:

Wild Game Enchiladas with a Chocolate Almond Mole Sauce 41

Tamale Cheese Pie with Double Smoked Quail 44

Entrees:

Macadamia Nut Crusted Red Snapper with a Mango Butter Sauce 47

Duck Breast with Red Chili Glaze 50

Mr. Pibb's Ribs with Sarsaparilla BBQ Sauce 52

Side Dishes:

Hominy and Green Bean Casserole 54

Mac N' Cheese 56

Dessert:

Tina Turner Mousse 58

Ibiza Restaurant. New Haven, Connecticut **Page 60**

Seared Salmon with Pistachio Vinaigrette and Catalan Style Spinach 61

Jean-Louis. Greenwich, Connecticut **Page 62**

Beef Cheeks Slowly Braised in Red Wine with Onion Compote and Foie Gras 63

Joel Brasserie. Atlanta, Georgia **Page 65**

Pommes Maxime (Thin Potato Crisps) 66

Croque Monsieur 67

La Bonne Auberge. New Hope, Pennsylvania **Page 68**

Potage Parmentier Leek and Potato Soup 69

La Piccola Liguria Ristorante. Port Washington, New York **Page 70**

Bow Tie Pasta a la Liguria 71

Nora. Washington, DC **Page 72**

Caesar Salad with Farm Fresh Eggs, Garlic Croutons & Parmesan 73

Chicken Breast with Goat Cheese & Walnut Stuffing 74

Potato Gratin 75

Fudgy Brownies 76

Park 75 at Four Seasons Hotel Atlanta. Atlanta, Georgia **Page 77**

Crab Mac-n-Cheese 78

Plaza Café. Southampton, New York **Page 79**

Chocolate Bread Pudding with Caramelized Bananas and Peanut Butter Ice Cream 79

Ristorante Café Cortina. Farmington Hills, Michigan **Page 82**

Zabaglione Mediterreano 83

Gnocchetti Di Casea Con Le Medaglioni Di Aragosta 84

Six89. Carbondale, Colorado **Page 85**

Lobster Corn Chowder 86

White Chocolate Chip Brownies 87

Solaris Grille. Center Square, Pennsylvania **Page 88**

House Penne 89

Splendido at The Chateau. Beaver Creek, Colorado **Page 90**

Mashed Potatoes 91

Spendido's Spicy Pecans 92

Potato Gnocchi, Toasted Garlic, Tomato, Basil and Guanciale 93

Lemon Blueberry Soufflé 95

Sweet Basil. Needham, Massachusetts **Page 98**

Rigatoni with Chicken, Broccoli, and Parmesan Cheese 99

Vie. Western Springs, Illinois **Page 100**

Almond Butter Cake 101

Vidalia. Washington, DC **Page 102**

Slow Cooked Vidalia Onions 102

The West End Grill. Ann Arbor, Michigan **Page 104**

Southwestern Crab Cakes 105

York Street. Dallas, Texas **Page 106**

D*MN Good Brownies 107

Chocolate Soup 108

Z Cuisine French Bistrot. Denver, Colorado **Page 109**

ColoRouge Tartiflette Fondue 110

Zingerman's. Ann Arbor, Michigan **Page 112**

Bluefish-Fried in Bacon with Blue Grits 113

Hangtown Fry 115

Chocolate and Bacon Fat Gravy 117

Chapter 6: Friendly Calories from Family and Friends Page 119

Appetizers: Page 119

Cocktail Meatballs 119

Hot Spinach/Cheese Salsa Quiche 120

Pesto and Sun Dried Tomato Torte 121

Beef Nachos Supreme 122

Main Dishes: Page 124

Baked Macaroni and Cheese 124

Blintz Soufflé 125

Bourek 126

Chicken Alfredo 127

Chicken, Zucchini and Avocado Tortillas 128

French Salisbury Steak with Garlic Cheese Toasts 129

French Toast Casserole 131

Individual Pizzas (Plain, Chicken, Pepperoni, Sausage Variations) 132

Linguine with Tomatoes and Basil 133

Mac & Cheese Recipe 134

Noodle/Spinach Casserole 135

Pasta with Sausage in Tomato Cream Sauce 136

Sharon's Dairy Kugel 137

Shepherd's Pie 138

String Pie 139

The Ultimate Grilled Cheese Sandwich 140

Side Dishes: Page 141

Broccoli Casserole 141

Cream of Spinach 142

Cream Soups (Asparagus, Broccoli, Celery, Corn, Mushrooms, Mushroom and Potato, Potato, Spinach, Tomato Variations) 143

Exotic Salad 145

Layered Lettuce 146

Mozzarella Sticks 147

Orzo and Scallion Pilaf 148

Pumpkin Soup 149

Potato Pancakes 150

Desserts: Page 151

Almond Candy Cookies 151
Apple Cobbler Pie 152
Baked Custard 153
Banana Bread with Chocolate Chips 154
Black Bottom Cupcakes 155
Carrot Cake 156
Chocolate Brownies 158
Chocolate Chip Cheesecake 159
Date Almond Delight 160
Devil Dog Recipe 161
Fruit Cobbler 162
Mississippi Mud or Dirt Pie 163
Pumpkin Tiramisu 165
Watermelon Nut Delight 166
12 East Cheesecake 169

Chapter 7: Calorie Rich Drinks Page 171

Ice Cream or Cold Energy Drinks Page 172

Apple Pie a La Mode 172
Black and White Milk Shake 172
Boost® Apricot Peach Smoothie 172
Boost® Blueberry Blast 173
Boost® Chocolate Coconut Delight 173
Boost® Creamy Pina Colada 173
Boost® Fuzzy Navel 173
Boost® Guava Banana 174
Boost® Mango Tango 174
Boost® Nutty Butter Banana Shake 174
Boost® PB & J Milkshake 174
Boost® Peach Perfection 175
Boost® Pumpkin Nog 175
Boost® Strawberry Banana 175
Chocolate Milk Shake 175
Chocolate-Peanut Butter Shake 176
Coco Coco Shake 176
Creamsicle 176
Great Grape Slush 176
High Calorie Carnation Shake 177
Ice Coffee 177
Orange Sherbet Shake 177
Peaches and Cream 177
Raspberry 178
Root Beer Float 178
Scandi Appleberry Punch 178
Scandi Banana Shake 178
Scandi Coconut Cider 179
Scandi Coconut Cream Pie 179
Scandi Cranorange Shake 179
Scandi Eggnog 179
Scandi Fruit Spritzer 180
Scandi Lemon Drop 180
Scandi Orange Creamsickle 180
Scandi Orange Julius 181
Scandi Peach Pie 181
Scandi Rasbery Twist 181

Scandi Strawberry Fields 182
Scandi Strawberry Fountain Shake 182
Strawberry Crush 182
Tropical Fruit Delight 183
Vanilla Milk Shake 183

Hot Drinks Page 184

Café Con Leche 184
Café Mocha 184
Cranberry Spiced Cider 184
Dulche de Leche 184
Emily's Banana Cream Pie 185
Heavenly Hot Chocolate 185
Hot Apple Cider 185
Hot Vanilla Not Chocolate 185
Oreos and Coconut Cream 186
Pumpkin Pie a La Talia 186

Introduction

Creative Calories & Recipes for Weight Gain is a different type of recipe book. It is a collaboration of a passion by a mother (of a child who lost excessive weight due to a struggle with anxiety) and two Registered Dietitians (RD's) who have learned over the years, that while there is an obesity epidemic occupying everyone's attention, there is an equally significant and under acknowledged problem on the other end of the spectrum, and that is malnutrition. In fact all three of us have learned through different work and life experiences, that being underweight and struggling to maintain or gain weight can be just as, if not more physically and emotionally difficult.

There are many reasons why people are underweight, ranging from genetics and/or psychological reasons to temporary or on-going medical conditions and diseases. It would be impossible to address any and every reason in this book. We hope to provide more general concepts, which will cover as many reasons as possible; however your specific situation may still require more individualization. In such cases, we encourage you to speak to your doctor and/or registered dietitian to work one-on-one with you in conjunction with this book, as appropriate. It is imperative that we emphasize that this recipe book is not intended for the general otherwise healthy person who is normal weight or overweight.

This book is intended for those who try/have tried desperately over the short-term or long-term to maintain and/or gain weight.

We struggled as registered dietitians with the idea that we would at times be possibly contradicting everything we and many others have learned and understood to be healthy eating. But again, it has been our experience with patients that has taught us (and anyone who has been through a similar experience) when a person is suffering from illness, pain, taste changes, depression, anxiety, etc. that interferes with his/her appetite and food intake, the goal is to fuel the body with calories, in certain cases *any* possible calories to avoid resorting to enteral and/or parenteral nutrition.* When all other options have been exhausted, it becomes a matter of what **can** or **will** someone eat, what will fuel their body, and providing just that. We see patients who for various and complex reasons, *can* only eat one or two foods. For a short while, it may be appropriate to give that patient only those one or two foods, permitting those one or two foods can actually provide adequate calories. Certainly a patient would require vitamin and mineral supplementation with such a limited food intake, but in these exceptional cases, calories are calories and the quality of the calories is not most important in such short-term cases. What is most important is ensuring this patient can maintain or gain weight.

Our book will of course offer many delicious recipes to help make it easier for you to enjoy eating and gaining weight, but in addition we will provide techniques, charts, and some lesser known secrets for increasing appetite and food intake. We offer heart healthy recipe substitutes for anyone who might need to follow such a plan for a longer period of time (more than 2-3 months) and particularly for those with a known family history of elevated cholesterol levels and/ or heart disease. If you are unsure whether or not you fall into this category, we encourage you to talk to your doctor before making changes to your diet. If you do have particular concerns regarding this, talking with your doctor and/ or registered dietitian is strongly recommended.

We hope you find the pages of this recipe book informative and helpful, but more importantly we hope that you find good food, support, hope, and health!

*There are medical situations when enteral and/or parenteral nutrition is an appropriate source of nutrition for a patient. Please work with your medical doctor regarding your particular situation.

Chapter 1 - First Things First about Weight Gain

Maximizing calorie consumption with every bite is important in promoting and maintaining weight gain. Remember that you need to eat more calories than you burn to gain weight; approximately 3,500 extra calories need to be consumed in order to gain approximately one pound. Caloric fortification of your regular recipes and frequent food consumption will help you add these needed calories. If able, eat at least 6 times a day starting off as 6 small meals and gradually increase to 3 larger meals and 3 substantial snacks. Again, everyone is different however and not everyone will be able to eat on such a specific schedule. It might take some trial and error to determine the best schedule to optimize calorie intake. It is also important to remember to consume liquids *after* snacks and meals instead of before or during.

Pick foods with concentrated calories for your snacks and meals. Avoid filling up on zero or low calorie liquids or foods. If you find that you get full easily, consume your liquids *after* your meal. Nuts, dried fruits, cheese and crackers, granola, guacamole and chips, peanut butter on crackers or fruit (apples or bananas), crackers or chips with sour cream or avocado based dips, puddings, custards, breads or biscuits spread with nut butters or olive oil, old fashioned milk shakes, and other high calorie drinks (see Chapter 7 for ideas) are all great "calorie dense" snack ideas for weight gain. Keep the food choices varied so you do not get bored or lose your taste for a favorite snack. Refer to Chapter 3 for more foods to keep on hand for high calorie snacking and meal preparation.

To increase calories, use nonfat dried milk in casseroles, meat loaf, lasagna, mashed potatoes and macaroni and cheese. Prepare hot cereals with evaporated or regular whole milk or even a little heavy cream. Instead of water add yogurt, evaporated milk, whole milk, heavy cream, grape juice or fruit nectars to blender drink recipes along with peanut butter, avocado (try it, it really is great and adds a lovely green hue), silken tofu, ice cream, fruit (canned or frozen in syrup), pie filling, apple butter, fruit purees, and/or sour cream.

Fortify your favorite recipes with additional calories by adding avocado, nuts, olives, olive oil, peanut butter, pre-cooked chopped meat, mashed beans, cheese, wheat germ, dried fruits or dried milk powder depending on whether you are preparing something sweet or savory. Always use milk instead of water when making scrambled eggs and coat the pan with oil and add cheese or cream cheese to increase the calories further. Cheese added to soup after it is served in individual bowls is another easy way to add calories as well as putting cheese sauce on fish, pasta, vegetables, meat or chicken. Adding calories is easy and fun. Experiment with the above suggestions to create new and exciting family favorites and send them to us at cravingcaloriesllc@gmail.com - perhaps we will post it on our website for everyone to try.

Remember Your Heart!

As mentioned in the introduction, we advise ensuring, particularly if there is a known family history of early heart disease in your family (i.e. heart attack or disease at, or before the age of 55) that you consult with a medical doctor and registered dietitian for additional guidance on gaining weight in a way that is intentionally heart healthy. What does this mean? It is actually possible to gain weight by eating food with *healthy* fats, such as olive and canola oil, nuts, or avocado to name a few. In fact some people have switched to such types of foods and fats in an effort to adopt a healthier lifestyle and **lose** weight, not realizing both good or healthy fats and bad or unhealthy fats (trans and saturated fats) still contain equal calories and therefore need to be limited for weight maintenance or weight loss. If you are trying to gain weight, this is a win-win situation for you! You are actually able and encouraged to eat more of these types of food (nuts, avocado, olive oil) to help you gain weight in a heart healthy way.

In this section we will provide tips on modifying any recipes in this book to create them in a heart healthy way by substituting certain ingredients for others. These substitutions have been time-tested and taste-tested and still result in delicious tasting foods and meals without concern about potentially increasing your cholesterol levels and damaging your heart health. This section is particularly important and strongly recommended if your effort to maintain or gain weight is on a more long-term basis. Happy heart-healthy eating!

Heart Healthy Recipe substitutions:

1 cup of butter (in baking)	1 cup applesauce or 1 cup canola or olive oil
8 ounces of cream cheese	8 ounces of nonfat or low fat yogurt or low fat or part-skim ricotta cheese
1 cup crème fraiche	1 cup nonfat or low fat yogurt or low fat or part-skim cheese
1 cup heavy cream (in recipes; not for whipping)	2 tsp cornstarch or 1 Tbsp flour whisked into 1 cup nonfat milk
1 cup sour cream	1 cup low-fat cottage cheese plus 2 Tbsp skim milk + 1 Tbsp lemon juice
1 cup fat or oil for sautéing	4 cups low fat stock, fruit juice or wine and sauté until liquid evaporates
1 egg	2 egg whites or egg substitutes (as per directions on package)
1 cup oil or fat for basting	1 cup fruit juice or low fat stock

Source: Linda Resnick and Dee Brock, *Food FAQs: Substitutions*, Yields & Equivalents, (2003, FAQs Press)

Weight Gain in Children

Weight gain in children can present unique challenges that are different from weight gain in adults. Consistent and appropriate calorie consumption in children is critical for growth and development. In addition, many children have a natural aversion to trying new foods (neophobia) and have limited food preferences. To optimize weight gain while supporting growth and development a varied/balanced diet is essential. Start by introducing new foods alongside personal favorites that have been fortified with extra calories. Optimize the calories in the foods your child already knows and enjoys by adding additional calories into your usual recipes to maximize the caloric content of their favorite foods. (See Chapter 3 for ideas). A child who happily eats macaroni and cheese will not notice that some extra butter/canola oil, non- fat dried milk or eggs have been added to their favorite recipe before cooking. Experiment by adding incremental amounts to create a fortified version of foods that they already love. Adding additional fats (butter, olive or canola oil, avocado slices, mayonnaise or salad dressings) to vegetables, pasta or sandwiches is another easy way to get more calories into someone with a small appetite. In addition, new high calorie foods can be introduced alongside their favorites as something that they can "try out". Although it will take more work and planning on your part and may not be accepted initially, after seeing it a few times it will no longer be new or scary for a child. By placing a new or "unknown" food next to the "known" food in the same meal or snack, you will avoid a situation where a new food needs to be consumed because it is the only thing that was prepared.

Snack foods are very important for weight gain and foods that are both nutrient and calorically dense should be emphasized. Common snacks that children typically eat tend to be processed low fiber carbohydrates that fill small stomachs easily, but do not provide all the macronutrients needed for growth and development. When you are feeding snacks to children, offer them foods that complement their favorite carbohydrate snacks in order to create a mini-meal. Graham crackers are great as the base for ricotta cheese, peanut or other nut butters (almond and cashew) but do not provide enough calories or nutrients by themselves. A child does not need to forgo the plain fish crackers, but a better choice would be a handful (child sized) of crackers supplemented by some mozzarella cheese along with some grapes, raisins or nuts and/or 4 ounces of 100% fruit juice, yogurt or milk to round it off. Providing high calorie dips like hummus, salad dressings, yogurt and guacamole make eating fruits, vegetables and carbohydrate foods more nutritious and fun! If you have a group of children, put each child's dip into their own bowl and let them dip as much as they like.

Offering a higher calorie version of foods that your child already eats is also beneficial. Whole, 2% or even 1% milk is a good choice for encouraging weight gain. If there is a strong family history of early heart disease (heart attack or disease at or before the age of 55) skim or soy milk that you fortify with non-fat dried milk powder or a little canola or mild olive oil will provide additional calories without adding saturated fat and skim milk with added protein (called "Skim Plus") is also available alongside the regular milk in the grocery store (refer to the Heart Healthy section within this chapter). Hot cocoa or oatmeal made with milk instead of water is another example of an easy way to add useful calories and nutrients as is using milk to thicken homemade or canned soups.

Please remember that these tips should supplement an already balanced diet that promotes and optimizes growth and development. We recommend speaking to a medical doctor or registered dietitian for an individualized nutrition evaluation and recommendations especially if your child has medical issues. Also it is important that a child's growth and development be monitored closely by your doctor or dietitian while incorporating such dietary changes. A growing body needs protein, carbohydrates, fats, vitamins, minerals and phytonutrients/phytochemicals (beneficial compounds that are not vitamins or minerals) that can only be provided by eating real food.

Lighting and Atmosphere: How it Affects Appetite!

If you stop and think about it, there is a reason why most five star restaurants have similar characteristics: dim lighting, soft, light music playing in the background, a comfortable, pleasing and relaxing atmosphere, not to mention delicious aromas filling the air, and waiters walking by with delicious-looking entrees on their trays. All of these factors actually encourage people to feel more hungry (increase appetite) and eat more food, often times more than they really need or want to. When trying to gain weight, we encourage you to consider the environment you typically eat in and as much as possible, to incorporate the following ideas and concepts. Believe it or not these concepts are equally if not more important in a hospital room. There is one very important consideration however. With certain medical conditions or therapies, a person's senses may be altered and what might ordinarily be considered a pleasing and enjoyable aroma or taste might have quite the opposite effect at that time. This will be very individual, and you need to determine what your likes and dislikes are in your particular situation and adjust them to suit your needs. But we encourage you to at least try, and hopefully you will find that some of these things work for you.

First, consider the dishes used to serve the food. Are they appealing? Do they make you feel special or as if you are out at a fancy restaurant or in the comfort of your own home? Start here, if your plates and dishware could be more appealing, make them that way, bring out the fancy china! Second, consider the overall atmosphere of the room. Consider putting a vase of flowers or a candle on the table, and/or add a table cloth. Think of how a nice white table cloth with nice place settings and a centerpiece can significantly change the atmosphere of a plain, drab cafeteria or hall. It is the same idea. Then, dim those lights! The lighting and atmosphere of a hospital room actually decrease appetite and make you eat less. Even research has shown that people eat more in dimly lit atmospheres. In addition, playing soft, classical or slow music can stimulate relaxation and appetite. If you are in a hospital, you may want to experiment with bringing in aromatic take-out food instead of eating the hospital food. You may also try non-burning scented candles; they make many delicious smelling scents which can help stimulate appetite. Remember again however, for some, aromas (even typically pleasing ones) can be irritating or nauseating depending on one's particular medical condition and/or therapy and it is important to be sensitive to that. In such cases try to minimize aromas and smells from food or cooking as much as possible. And last, but certainly not least consider what the food looks like. As much as possible, choose foods that look appetizing and do not forget about enhancing its presentation in ways described above.

Chapter 2 - Metabolism and Exercise

Metabolism or our body's ability to utilize energy in the form of calories is influenced by many things to a lesser or greater extent. Genetics is typically the biggest influence on metabolism, but additional factors such as body temperature regulation, fever, stress, illness, and/ or healing needs of the body can increase the basal metabolic rate of an individual. In addition, it is well known that exercise or physical activity increases metabolism. However, most people typically think about exercise for losing weight and burning calories. It is equally important to consider how physical activity or exercise throughout the day will affect your efforts to maintain or gain weight. One pound of body weight equals about 3,500 calories. Therefore, if you are trying to gain weight and want to gain one pound per week, you will need to increase your calorie intake by 500 calories per day each of the seven days in a week (500 calories x 7 days = 3,500 calories= one pound). Recent research has shown that this math while correct in the abstract sense may not be as exact on an individual basis. Use these numbers as guidelines to estimate the number of calories that you actually burn and if you are not gaining weight as you would like, you need to consume more or burn less calories. Consultation with a registered dietitian is recommended to help in such cases.

In addition to thinking about how many calories you need to eat, it is also critical to determine how many calories you burn through exercise and physical activity so that you can compensate for those. If you require 2,500 calories per day to gain weight, and you eat 2,500 on a given day, but bike for about 60 minutes, you will have burned about 375 calories, so you now have a caloric deficit of 375 calories, which means your total caloric intake for the day was really only about 2125 calories. Therefore to make up for the calories you burned or "lost," you will have to ensure that you replace those calories by eating more calories that day. We have included a convenient table and examples to make this easier for you to understand and adjust your own calories as needed based on your level of physical activity (See Exercise and Calorie information on the next page).

In addition to physical activity and exercise, your schedule of eating can influence how you "metabolize" calories. Eating more frequently will enable you to consume more calories. Aim for eating something every two hours and keep your meals high in calorie dense foods. There is no need to stick to mealtimes or even to regular meal foods in order to consume more calories. Be creative and eat what your body craves when you crave it.

Avoid things that are bulky that just fill you up but do not provide calories or nutrients. In addition if you have times during the day when you are hungrier or able to eat more food, take advantage of that and try to eat more. If you find that your appetite seems decreased or your stomach feels full often, do some mild exercise. Moving your body will stimulate your digestive tract and help to stimulate your appetite to help you consume more food.

Calorie Compensation

Based on 60 Minutes of Exercise and an average 150 lb person (adjust accordingly)
The following list displays the calories burned (expended) and two choices (fast food suggestion or other food suggestion) to compensate for the calories expended.

Exercise	Calories Expended	Fast Food Suggestion	Other Food Options
Jogging	450	Starbucks Cinnamon Roll (500 calories)	8 oz Greek style yogurt with ½ C Quaker Natural Granola (450 calories)
Brisk Walking (15 min/mile)	300	McDonald's® Egg McMuffin (300 calories)	12 oz. sweetened iced tea and Nature Valley® granola bar (300 calories)
Swimming (25 yards/minute)	360	Taco Bell Burrito Supreme, Beef (410 calories)	4 graham crackers with 2 Tbsp peanut butter and 4 oz 2% milk (360 calories)
Bicycling (6 minutes/mile)	376	Starbucks Grande 2% caramel Frappuccino with whipped crème (380 calories)	2 Buttermilk Biscuits with 2 Tbsp Jam (400 calories)
Tennis	480	Panera Chocolate Chipper (440 Calories)	1 cup Ben and Jerry's Chunky Monkey Ice Cream (480 calories)
Table Tennis	270	Dunkin Donuts Chocolate Frosted Donut (230 calories)	4 Oreo double stuff cookies (270 calories)
Soccer	584	Wendy's Large French Fries (540 calories)	3 oz cheddar cheese, 8 Ritz Crackers and 8 oz apricot nectar (590 calories)
Dancing (noncontact)	300	Pizza Hut Large Hand-Tossed Style Cheese Pizza (1 slice; 320 calories)	16 oz. Odwalla™ Mango Tango Smoothie (300 calories)
Skating (ice or roller)	600	Johnny Rockets Grilled Cheese Sandwich (520 calories)	1 C Ben and Jerry's Chubby Hubby ice cream (600 calories)

Exercise	Calories Expended	Fast Food Suggestion	Other Food Options
Light Housekeeping	270	Dunkin Donuts Chocolate Cream Filled Doughnut (310 calories)	Pepperidge Farm® Sausalito chocolate chunk cookie and 8 oz 2% milk (270 calories)
Gardening	270	½ Cup full-fat Vanilla Ice Cream (270 calories)	8 oz grape juice and 1 oz Pepperidge Farm® cheese goldfish (270 calories)
Hiking (no load)	464	El Pollo Loco Cheese Quesadilla (495 calories)	1/3 C mixed nuts, 1/3 C dried fruit and 8 oz flavored sports drink (464 calories)
Skiing	390	Cinnabon cinnamon Stick (379 calories)	Hot chocolate and a glazed doughnut (390 calories)
Cross country Skiing (leisurely)	464	Subway® 6 inch tuna sandwich (464 calories)	1 Cup chocolate pudding made with 2% milk and 2 Pepperidge Farm® Shortbread cookies
Snow Shoeing (soft snow)	680	Johnny Rocket's Cheese Fries (760 calories)	12 oz hot chocolate and a peanut butter (2 Tbsp) and jelly (1 Tbsp) sandwich (740 calories) or French fries with melted cheese (678 calories)
Aerobic Exercise (low impact)	344	Starbucks Grande 2% Tazo® Green Tea Latte (350 calories)	1/3 C guacamole and 18 Tortilla chips (350 calories)
Raking leaves	224	Dunkin Donuts White Hot Chocolate small (230 calories)	8 oz low fat fruit yogurt (10 grams protein/cup) (224 calories)
Weight Training (40 seconds between sets)	714	Burger King® Original Whopper With Cheese (770 calories)	16 oz. Odwalla™ Protein Smoothie vanilla (714 calories)
Volleyball (game)	360	Au Bon Pain Chocolate Chip Brownie (380 calories)	Carnation® Breakfast Essentials™ Chocolate prepared with 2% milk and 4 graham crackers (360 calories)
Basketball (game)	660	Dunkin Donuts Chipotle Chicken Sandwich (600 calories)	5 buttermilk pancakes and ¼ cup syrup (660 calories)

Adapted from:
www.nutribase.com and *Exercise Physiology* by William McArdle, Frank Katch, and Victor Katch, 1986 Lea and Febiger Publishers, Philadelphia.
Starbucks website: www.starbucks.com
Odwalla™ website: www.odwalla.com
Yahoo Fresh Picks by Sarah Fuss: http://food.yahoo.com/blog/yahoo freshpicks/9960/what-chain-food-favorites-cost-in-exercise "What Chain-Food Favorites Cost in Exercise," Posted Mon, Jun 01, 2009, 12:42 pm PDT.

Chapter 3 - Convenient Calories and Calorie Boosters

Keep on Hand To Add Calories and Nutrients

Non-perishables	Refrigerated Items	Frozen Foods
Apricot Nectar	Cheeses	Coconut ice cream
Avocados	Cream Cheese	Frozen Cookie Doughs
Baby food fruit and vegetable purees	Eggs	Frozen Fruit (in syrup if available)
Canned Chicken	Fruit Smoothie drinks	Frozen Fruit Concentrates
Canned Creamed Corn	Ground Turkey, Chicken, Beef, Pork, Lamb	Frozen Pesto
Canned Salmon	Heavy Cream	Frozen Pie Crusts
Canned Tuna	Nuts and Nut Butters	Frozen Pizza Dough
Canola Oil	Olives (black, green, pitted, with pits, sliced and whole)	Frozen Puff Pastry
Chocolate	Omega-3 Rich Spread	Frozen Waffles
Chocolate Hazelnut Spread	Pesto	Ice Cream
Coconut Milk	Ricotta Cheese	Sherbet
Condensed Milk	Sour Cream	Sorbet
Crackers	Soy Milk	
Dried Coconut	Tapenade (olive spread)	
Dried Fruit	Tofu (silken for shakes and sauces, soft for adding to casseroles)	
Fruit canned in juice/syrup	Yogurt Drinks	
Fruit Purees	Yogurt (2% or Whole)	
Granola	Whipped Cream	
Granola Bars	Whole Milk	
Grape Juice (white or purple)		
Nonfat Dried Milk		
Nuts		
Olive Oil		
Peanuts		
Peanut Butter		
Raisin Bread		

Chapter 4 - Fast and Furious Calories

Fast Food Items With 700+ Calories

While fast food restaurants typically have a bad reputation for anyone who is trying to lose weight, we find that there certainly can be a time and place for them when you are trying to gain weight. Fast and furious calories are quick and convenient calories, usually in a relatively small volume of food, technically referred to as "calorically-dense" foods. We do not recommend relying exclusively or even predominantly on fast-foods for weight gain, but we know when you are in a hurry with no time to cook, and you are craving calories, these fast-foods can be very convenient and they "get the job done." For such times, we have provided some examples of the *most* fast and furious calories around the nation.

Top Calorie-Packed Meals by Restaurant

A&W	Original Bacon Double Cheeseburger Calories: **800**		
Arby's	Meatball Toasted Sub Calories: **1000**	Arby's Mozzarella Sticks - Large (8) Calories: **849**	Arby's Chicken Parmesan Toasted Sub Calories**: 843**
Boston Market	Sirloin Dip Carver Calories: **1000**	Meatloaf Carver Calories: **940**	Pastry Top Chicken Pot Pie Calories: **780**
Burger King®	Triple Whopper Sandwich With Cheese Calories: **1230**	Quad Stacker Calories: **1000**	Double Whopper Sandwich with Cheese Calories: **990**
Carl's	Jr® Double Six Dollar Burger Calories: **1520**	Jr® Bacon Cheese Six Dollar Burger Calories: **1070**	Jr® Double Western Bacon Cheeseburger Calories: **970**
Dairy Queen®	Chicken Strip Basket (6 piece) Calories: **1270**	Dairy Queen Flame Thrower GrillBurger (1/2 lb) Calories: **1030**	Dairy Queen Chicken Strip Basket (4 piece) Calories: **1030**
Del Taco	Macho Nachos Calories: **1100**	Macho Combo Burrito Calories: **1050**	Macho Bacon & Egg Burrito Calories: **1030**
Dunkin Donuts	Sausage Egg Cheese Biscuit Sandwich Calories: **800**	Pastrami Supreme Sandwich Calories: **760**	

Hardee's®	Double Thickburger Calories: **1250**	Six Dollar Burger Calories: **1060**	Big Country Breakfast Platter – Sausage Calories: **1060**
Jack In The Box	Fish & Chips (Large) Calories: **830**	Sirloin Steak 'n' Cheddar Ciabatta Calories: **770**	Sourdough Jack Calories: **710**
KFC	Chicken and Biscuit Bowl™ Calories: **870**	Chicken Pot Pie Calories: **770**	
McDonald's®	Double Quarter Pounder with Cheese Calories: **740**	Big Breakfast (Large Size Biscuit) Calories: **790**	Big Breakfast (Regular Size Biscuit) Calories: **720**
Nathan's	Fish N Chips Calories: **1537**	Nathan's Chicken Tender Platter Calories: **1300**	Nathan's French Fries (Super Size) Calories: **1188**
Pizza Hut	Meat Lover's® 6" Personal Pan Pizza (whole pizza) Calories: **890**	Pizza Hut Supreme 6" Personal Pan Pizza (whole pizza) Calories: **710**	
Sonic	Super Sonic Cheeseburger (with mayo) Calories: **980**	Fritos Chili Pie Calories: **940** Or Chicken Strip Dinner (4) Calories: **930**	Super Sonic Cheeseburger (with ketchup) Calories: **900**
Subway®	Double Meatball Marinara Calories: **860**	8" Pizza (Sausage) Calories: **830**	8" Pizza (Pepperoni) Calories: **790**
Taco Bell®	Fiesta Taco Salad Calories: **840**	Taco Bell Nachos BellGrande Calories: **770**	
Wendy's®	Baconator Calories: **830**	Double w/Everything and Cheese Calories: **700**	
White Castle	Chicken Rings (20) Calories: **1130**	White Castle Fish Nibblers (sack) Calories: **1090**	White Castle Onion Chips (sack) Calories: **980**

Fast Food Drinks With 700+ Calories

Top Calorie-Packed Shakes and Drinks by Restaurant

A&W	M&M Polar Swirl (medium) Calories: **710**	Reese's Polar Swirl (medium) Calories: **740**	Vanilla Milkshake (medium) Calories: **720**
Burger King®	Chocolate Milk Shake - Large Calories: **950**	Oreo Sundae Shake - Strawberry - Medium Calories: **940**	Strawberry Milk Shake - Large Calories: **930**
Carl's	Jr® Oreo Cookie Shake Calories: **720**	Carl's Jr® Oreo Cookie Malt Calories: **790**	Carl's Jr® Vanilla Malt Calories: **780**
Chic-Fil-A'	Hand-Spun Milkshake (Chocolate) Calories: **760**	Hand-Spun Milkshake (Cookies & Cream) Calories: **790**	Hand-Spun Milkshake (Strawberry) Calories: **730**
Dairy Queen®	Large Choc. Chip Cookie Dough Blizzard Calories: **1320**	Large Chocolate Malt Calories: **1300**	Large Chocolate Shake Calories: **1130**
Dunkin Donuts	Tropical Fruit Smoothie (Large) Calories: **720**		
Hardee's®	Hardee's Chocolate Malt (Hand-Dipped) Calories: **780**	Hardee's Strawberry Malt (Hand-Dipped) Calories: **775**	Hardee's Vanilla Malt (Hand-Dipped) Calories: **770**
Jack In The Box	Oreo Cookie Ice Cream Shake – 16 oz Calories: **910**	Jack In The Box Oreo Cookie Ice Cream Shake (24 oz) Calories: **1290**	Jack In The Box Chocolate Ice Cream Shake (24 oz) Calories: **1230**

McDonald's®	Chocolate Triple Thick Shake (32 oz) Calories: **1160**	Vanilla Triple Thick Shake (32 oz) Calories: **1110**	Strawberry Triple Thick Shake (32 oz) Calories: **1110**
Sonic	Peanut Butter Shake - Large (20 oz) Calories: **1010**	Chocolate Cream Pie Shake - Large (20 oz) Calories: **990**	Peanut Butter Fudge Shake- Large (20 oz) Calories: **940**
Sonic	Strawberry Cream Pie Shake - Large (20 oz) Calories: **930**	M&M's Sonic Blast - Large (20 oz) Calories: **900**	
White Castle	Chocolate Shake – Large Calories by Region: (**1680** Louisville) (**1230** New Jersey) (**1130** Cincinnati) (**1090** Nashville) (**1020** New York) (**950** St Louis) (**890** Columbus & Detroit)	Vanilla Shake – Large Calories by Region: (**1180** New Jersey) (**1140** Cincinnati) (**1090** Nashville) (**990** New York) (**940** Minneapolis) (**860** Columbus & Detroit)	Strawberry Shake – Large Calories by Region: (**1090** Minneapolis) (**1010** Columbus & Detroit) (**840** Cincinnati) (**830** Chicago) (**790** Minneapolis)

Restaurants, food items outlined, and their calorie count may vary as products/ ingredients may change.

Chapter 5 - Distinguished Calories from Distinguished Chefs

This chapter includes over 50 delicious recipes from top rated chefs located throughout the United States. Each chef created special high calorie recipes/menus or provided us with customer favorites for this cookbook.

A SPECIAL THANK YOU TO THE CHEFS FROM THE FOLLOWING RESTAURANTS. . ...

Arpeggio. Springhouse, Pennsylvania... **Bayona**. New Orleans, Louisiana...**California School of Culinary Art**. Los Angeles, California...**Carlos Restaurant**. Highland Park, Illinois... **Charlie Trotter's**. Chicago, Illinois...**Michel Richard Citronelle**. Washington, DC...**Dante & Luigi's Corona di ferro**. Philadelphia, Pennsylvania...**Hudson's on the Bend**. Austin, Texas...**Ibiza** Restaurant. New Haven, Connecticut...**Jean-Louis**. Greenwich, Connecticut...**Joel Brasserie**. Atlanta, Georgia...

La Bonne Auberge. New Hope, Pennsylvania...**La Piccola Liguria Ristorante**. Port Washington, New York...

Park 75 at Four Seasons Hotel Atlanta. Atlanta, Georgia...**Plaza Café**. Southampton, New York...**Nora**. Washington, DC...**Ristorante Café Cortina**. Farmington Hills, Michigan...**Six89**. Carbondale, Colorado...**Solaris Grille**. Center Square, Pennsylvania...**Splendido at The Chateau**. Beaver Creek, Colorado...**Sweet Basil**. Needham, Massachusetts...**Vie**. Western Springs, Illinois...**Vidalia. An American Restaurant & Bar**. Washington, DC...**The West End Grill**. Ann Arbor, Michigan...**York Street**. Dallas, Texas...**Z Cuisine French Bistrot**. Denver, Colorado...**Zingerman's**. Ann Arbor, Michigan

Arpeggio

Springhouse, Pennsylvania

Contributed by: Mary, Co-Owner

Mediterranean Mini Crustless Quiche

Recipe Anecdotes

Mini Quiches: We usually have a long line on Friday nights, so we offer food while waiting. Sometimes we hand out pizza, but Friday is pizza night so I wanted to develop something that would not involve that station. These mini quiches are easy to make and easy to eat and are a favorite among our customers!

Total Time: 30 Minutes

Ingredients:

2 eggs and 1 egg white

4 oz feta cheese, crumbled

20 Kalamata olives pitted and finely diced

Pepper to taste

Directions:

Mix ingredients together

Grease mini muffin tins

Fill each tin about ¾ full and bake at 350° F for 20 minutes

Cool 5 minutes, flip over to unmold and serve immediately

Recipe makes 24 servings of mini quiches. All values are per serving. **Calories: 93,** Protein: 2, Total Fat: 9, Saturated Fat: 5

Chocolate Bread Pudding (Molten Center) Topped with Caramelized Bananas

Recipe Anecdotes

Bread Pudding has become a staple at Arpeggio, and we have become well known for it! The basic recipe for bread pudding was given to me in Atlanta many years ago by my chef sister in law, Lynne Gigliotti (AKA Chef G at the CIA in Hyde Park) who is responsible for my culinary inspiration and much of my education over the years. This is one of many variations created with her original recipe, and is a winter favorite at the restaurant.

Total Time: 65–85 minutes

Ingredients:

1 quart hard crusted bread cubed

1 quart heavy cream

12 ounce semi sweet chocolate

1 cup sugar

12 eggs

¼ cup vanilla extract

12 one ounce squares semi sweet chocolate

9 X 12 inch baking pan

6 - 8 bananas sliced

2 TBSP butter

½ cup brown sugar

Directions:

Prepare the following and soak for several hours or overnight:

Melt 12 oz chocolate with ½ qt heavy cream in double boiler over medium heat

Wisk occasionally while melting

Remove top pan and cool for 15-20 minutes

While this is cooling, whisk together the other ½ qt cream, 1 C sugar, eggs, vanilla

When cooled, slowly whisk chocolate mixture into egg mixture (Hint: Make sure it is cool enough and that you pour slowly enough or eggs will curdle!)

Add cubed bread and soak for several hours or overnight

When you are ready to Bake

Preheat oven to 350° F

Spray baking pan with PAM and pour mixture into pan

Divide pan into 12 by eye and place 1 square of chocolate lengthwise into the middle of each serving

Place in the middle of the oven and reduce temperature to 300° F

Bake approximately 45-50 minutes and cool for 1 hour

To make topping:

Slice the bananas.

Melt the butter in a skillet on medium heat and then add the bananas

Sprinkle with sugar and sauté the bananas until golden

Cut the bread pudding into 12 servings, top with warm bananas and enjoy!

Make ahead option:

This bread pudding can be made ahead and refrigerated

You can reheat it in the microwave if refrigerated; if frozen, it must be fully defrosted before microwaving by placing in the refrigerator for a full day.

Recipe makes 12 servings. All values are per serving. **Calories: 822**, Protein: 12g, Total Fat: 56g, Sat. Fat: 33g

Medjool Dates Stuffed with Mascarpone Cheese and Walnuts

Recipe Anecdotes

Dates: The dates were developed for my kitchen chefs at the restaurant to thank them for their great work! The stuffed dates are on the top of their request list!

Total Time: 30 minutes

Ingredients:

20 Dates

Stuffing:

½ pound mascarpone or cream cheese

4 Tbsp confectioner sugar

½ cup toasted walnut pieces

Dash of orange oil

Dash of vanilla extract

Directions:

Pit dates

Slice one side of each date lengthwise

Press ends and remove seed with small spoon or tweezers

Mix stuffing ingredients

Fill ingredients with small demitasse spoon and press to close date. (optional: they can also be sliced in half)

Sprinkle lightly with cinnamon before serving.

Recipe makes 20 dates. All values are per serving. **Calories: 130**, Protein: 2, Total Fat: 6, Saturated Fat: 3

Bayona

New Orleans, Louisiana

Contributed by: Susan Spicer

Restaurant Anecdotes

Bayona is located in a 200-year-old Creole cottage in the heart of the romantic French Quarter. The main dining area is comprised of 3 rooms, each slightly different in décor, but all with a warm, comfortable ambiance. Terra cotta-colored walls, dark green, faux marble accents, huge hand-colored photographs of Italian gardens and trompe l'oeil.

Mediterranean landscapes are some of the design elements that lend an elegant, European feel. The lush courtyard with fountains is ideal for outdoor dining in spring and fall.

There is also a charming, private dining room upstairs for parties of 16-30. The service staff is knowledgeable, friendly and efficient. The award-winning wine list offers over 400 selections from around the world.

Smoked Duck Hash with Calvados Sauce

Total Time: If all Prep Work is completed, it will take 15 - 20 minutes

Ingredients:

1lb Puff Pastry, rolled out & cut into 12 4" squares

2 Tbsp Butter

¼ cup Onion Dice (1/4")

¼ cup Celery Dice

¼ cup Andouille Sausage Dice

1 cup Green Apple Dice

1 cup Smoked Duck Meat, Diced

¼ cup Cooked Sweet Potato Dice

3 Tbsp Flour

2 Tbsp Sherry

1 cup Chicken Broth

1 tsp each chopped Sage and Thyme, preferably fresh

Salt and Pepper

Directions:

Melt butter in sauté pan.

When bubbling, add onion and celery dice and cook for 2 minutes, then add andouille and apple.

Turn up the heat and cook for 2 more minutes, then add smoked duck and sweet potato.

Stir and sprinkle with flour.

Cook for 1 minute; then add sherry and half of the chicken broth, stirring to mix.

Bring to a boil, and if mixture is too dry, add the rest of the broth.

Add herbs and taste for seasoning. The mixture should be moist but not too wet.

Cook for about 2 more minutes; then remove from heat and allow to cool.

Preparation:

1 lb Puff Pastry, rolled out and cut into 12" squares

1 Egg, beaten with 2 Tbsp milk.

Brush edges of chilled pastry square lightly with egg wash.

Place 3 oz (about 1/12) of the filling in the center of the square and bring two opposite corners of the square to meet in the center.

Then bring the other two corners to the center to form a small pyramid and pinch the 4 seams to seal.

Brush lightly with egg and refrigerate.

Ingredients for Calvados Sauce:

2 Shallots, minced

1 cup Apple Juice

¼ cup Apple Cider Vinegar

2 cups Veal Stock or Stock made from Smoked Duck

1 Tbsp Apple Jelly

2 Tbsp Calvados

Directions:

Combine first 4 ingredients in small pot.
Bring to a boil and reduce to 1 cup.
Whisk in jelly and Calvados and boil for about 2 minutes, or until mixture is slightly syrupy.
Keep warm, but not hot

To Serve:

Preheat oven to 450° F

Bake hashes packets for 12 minutes and serve with Calvados Sauce

Recipe makes 12 packets. All values are per packet. **Calories: 298**, Protein: 6g, Total Fat: 17g, Saturated Fat: 5g

California School of Culinary Art

Los Angeles, California

Contributed By: Chef Jon Beskow

JB's Cajun Potato Salad

Total Time: 40 Minutes plus time to cool if desired

<u>Ingredients</u>: **1** ½ lbs New Potato/Red Potato

¾ cup Celery

¾ cup Green Bell Pepper

¾ cup Onion, Yellow

1 each Garlic Clove, Minced

¼ Pound Bacon, Cut into Strips

½ cup Mayonnaise

2 tsp Tabasco

2 tsp Salt

2 tsp Pepper

As needed Butter

<u>Directions</u>:

Cut the pepper, onion and celery into ½" by ½" squares. Sauté them in butter as needed until almost translucent and then add the garlic and cook till translucent. Set aside to cool

Bring a pot of water to a simmer. Simmer potatoes whole until just tender. Once cooked through, remove the potatoes and cool.
In a sauté pan, add the bacon and cook until crispy. Remove from the pan to paper towels and drain.

Cut the potatoes into quarters and place in a mixing bowl. Add the sautéed vegetables, bacon, and mayonnaise to the bowl and fold gently until combined.

Season with salt, pepper, and Tabasco. The Tabasco or lemon juice can also be used to thin out the mayonnaise if the salad is too thick.

Recipe makes 8 Servings. All values are per serving. **<u>Calories: 304</u>**, Protein: 8g, Total Fat: 21g , Saturated Fat: 6g

CARLOS'
RESTAURANT

Highland Park, Illinois

Contributed by: Toni Gramm

Restaurant Anecdotes

Debbie and Carlos Nieto opened their restaurant, Carlos' in November of 1981. From the start, Carlos' has received many accolades from the Chicago Tribune, Chicago Magazine, Chicago Sun-Times, North Shore Magazine and Food and Wines' Top 25 restaurants in North America.

Rated number-one in the Chicago-area food rankings by *Zagat* with a nearly perfect "Food" score of 29 out of 30, Carlos' has been voted by "Gourmet" Magazine as a top restaurant.

The restaurant has been awarded the Wine Spectator's Grand Award for its winning wine list since 1990.

Hands-on, husband-and-wife owners Carlos and Debbie Nieto are excited to showcase their accomplishments with special events, and numerous memorable culinary evenings. Considered one of the oldest and best fine-dining options in the Chicago area.

Mushroom Crusted Petit Filet Mignon with Butter Poached Fingerling Potatoes, Broccoli Raab and a Cabernet-Mushroom Reduction

Total Time: 35 minutes

Ingredients:

6 Filet Mignon (6 ounces each) rolled in

2 cups finely chopped mushrooms

Grill in 450° F oven or on the barbeque for 6 – 10 minutes per side depending on desired degree of cooking

Ingredients Fingerling Potatoes:

1 ½ lbs Fingerling Potatoes (cut in half lengthwise)

Bay leaf, peppercorn and thyme

4 cups butter (clarified)

Directions to make Fingerling Potatoes:

Combine potatoes, bay leaf, peppercorn, and thyme with clarified butter and cook over low heat until potatoes are soft.

Strain and keep warm, season with salt and pepper

Directions for Broccoli Raab:

Blanch and shock

Ingredients for caramelized onions:

2 cups Pearl Onions

1 Tbsp sugar

1 cup white wine

2 Tbsp butter

Directions for caramelized onions:

Caramelize onions in sugar, white wine and butter

Ingredients for Cabernet Mushroom Reduction:

4 cups Mushrooms (small diced)

2 Tbsp butter

2 cups Mushroom Stock

3 cups Red Wine

1 cup Demi-glaze

1 Tbsp sugar

Salt and Pepper to taste

Directions to make Cabernet-Mushroom Reduction:

Caramelize Mushroom in a little butter and deglaze with mushroom stock.

Reduce by half and add red wine.

Add a tablespoon of sugar and reduce by half.

Strain and add to demi-glaze and reduce until desired thickness

Serve filet mignon with Cabernet-Mushroom reduction, caramelized onions, broccoli raab and fingerling potatoes

Recipe makes 6 servings. All values are per serving. **Calories: 967,** Protein: 56 g, Total Fat: 64 g, Saturated Fat: 29 g

Charlie Trotter's

Chicago, Illinois

Contributed By: Chef Charlie Trotter

BACKGROUND

July 2009 - Charlie Trotter's is regarded as one of the finest restaurants in the world. For nearly 22 years, the restaurant has dedicated itself to excellence in the culinary arts. The restaurant is recognized by many prestigious national and international institutions, including Relais & Chateaux and Traditions & Qualité. Among its many awards include Five Stars from the Mobil Travel Guide, Five Diamonds by AAA and ten James Beard Foundation awards, including 'Outstanding Restaurant' (2000) and 'Outstanding Chef' (1999).

Wine Spectator named the restaurant, 'The Best Restaurant in the World for Wine & Food' (1998) and 'America's Best Restaurant' (2000). Chef Trotter is the author of 14 cookbooks, three management books, and is the host of the nationally aired, award winning PBS cooking series, The Kitchen Sessions with Charlie Trotter. In addition to Charlie Trotter's, he also owns and operates the Michelin 1 Star Restaurant Charlie and Bar Charlie in the Palazzo Hotel, Casino & Resort in Las Vegas, and Trotter's To Go gourmet retail shop in Chicago.

Beyond his numerous culinary accolades, Chef Trotter has many philanthropic ties to a vast number of charities. Closest to his heart is the Charlie Trotter Culinary Education Foundation, which to date has raised over a million dollars.

Chef Trotter has received awards at the White House from both President Bush and Colin Powell for his work with his Culinary Foundation and was named one of only five 'heroes' to be honored by Colin Powell's charity, Americas Promise. In 2005, Chef Trotter was awarded the Humanitarian of the Year award by the International Association of Culinary Professionals for his overall service to the community.

Future corporate plans include opening a new restaurant in the Flatiron district of New York City as well as a retrospective cookbook reflecting the evolution of his culinary style over the past 15 years.

Goat Cheese and Basil Ravioli with Tomato Water

Total Time: 30 minutes plus 8 hours for Tomato Water preparation. Note: ravioli can be prepared ahead

<u>Ingredients</u> for Tomato Water:

10 Beefsteak tomatoes, chopped

Salt and freshly ground black pepper

<u>Ingredients</u> for Ravioli:

4 ounces soft goat cheese

2 Tbsp chopped fresh basil

2 Tbsp minced shallots

2 Tbsp chopped fresh chives

Salt and freshly ground black pepper

32 3-inch square wonton skins

1 egg slightly beaten

12 red teardrop tomatoes, peeled and blanched

4 yellow teardrop tomatoes, peeled and blanched

1 Tbsp tiny red basil shoots

1 Tbsp tiny green basil shoots

<u>Directions</u> to Prepare the Tomato Water:

Puree the tomatoes and season with salt.

Pour the puree into a cheesecloth-lined sieve set in a large bowl and refrigerate for 8 hours, or until all of the juices have dropped from the puree

Discard the solids from the tomato puree and place the tomato water in a small saucepan.

Cook over medium heat for 5 to 7 minutes, or until warm.

Season to taste with salt and pepper

Directions to Prepare the Ravioli Filling:

Place the goat cheese, chopped basil, shallots, and chives in a medium bowl and mix until combined

Season to taste with salt and pepper

Directions to Prepare the Ravioli:

Bring a pot of salted water to a boil

Place a wonton skin on a flat work surface and spoon 1 tablespoon of the filling in the center

Lightly brush the edges with the egg and top with another wonton skin.

Firmly press the edges of the wontons to seal

Repeat the process with the remaining ingredients (The ravioli can be prepared to this point several hours in advance and refrigerated on a floured sheet pan.)

Cook the ravioli in the boiling water for 3 minutes, or until al dente, then drain.

Place 4 ravioli in each shallow bowl and ladle 3 red tomatoes, 1 yellow tomato and tomato water over each bowl.

Sprinkle red and green basil shoots over the ravioli and top with freshly ground black pepper.

Recipe makes 4 servings. All values are per serving. **Calories: 292**, Protein: 14 g, Total Fat: 8.3, Saturated Fat: 4.7

Rack of Lamb with Crispy Polenta and Mustard Sauce

Total Time: 50 Minutes plus Overnight Marination

Ingredients:

The Lamb

2 Trimmed racks of lamb (about two pounds each)

5 Tbsp extra virgin olive oil

3 Tbsp chopped mixed fresh herbs (rosemary, thyme, and/or marjoram, in any combination)

Salt and freshly ground black pepper

Directions:

To Marinate the Lamb

Rub the lamb with 3 tablespoons of the olive oil, sprinkle with 2 tablespoons of the herbs, and marinate overnight.

To Cook the Lamb

Preheat the oven to 450°.

Heat a large ovenproof pan over medium-high heat, add the remaining 2 tablespoons olive oil, and sear the lamb on all sides.

Roast in the oven for 8 to 12 minutes, or until slightly less than the desired degree of doneness.

Remove the pan from the oven and allow the lamb to rest for 5 minutes.

Slice each rack between the bones just prior to serving, and season to taste with salt and pepper.

Reserve the lamb juices.

Polenta

1½ cups water

½ cup polenta

¼ cup roasted garlic cloves with the cooking oil

3 Tbsp unsalted butter

Salt and freshly ground black pepper

To Prepare the Polenta

Bring the water to a boil in a medium saucepan and slowly add the polenta.

Simmer over low heat, stirring occasionally, for 30 minutes, or until done.

Puree the roasted garlic with the cooking oil until smooth.

Mix 2 tablespoons of the butter and all of the garlic into the polenta and season to taste with salt and pepper.

Spread the mixture into a plastic wrap-lined 8-inch square pan and refrigerate for 2 hours.

To Cook the Polenta

Cut the polenta into four 3-inch circles.

Cook the polenta in the remaining 1 tablespoon butter in a medium sauté pan over medium-high heat for 3 minutes on each side, or until golden brown and crispy.

Mustard Sauce

¼ cup Dijon mustard

2 Tbsp white wine

1/3 cup lamb cooking juices

1 tablespoon fresh baby soft thyme

To Prepare the Mustard Sauce

Combine the mustard, white wine, and lamb juices in a bowl.

Whisk until well blended

Garnish

1 Tbsp fresh baby soft thyme

To Serve

Place a crispy polenta circle in the center of each plate.

Arrange the cut lamb racks on one edge of the polenta, and spoon the sauce around the plates.

Garnish with baby thyme.

Recipe makes 4 Servings. All values are per serving. **Calories: 1125**, Protein: 55 g, Total Fat: 92 g, Saturated Fat: 33 g

MICHEL RICHARD
CITRONELLE

Washington, DC

Contributed By: Chef Michel Richard

Restaurant Anecdotes

Michel Richard Citronelle, is a celebration of the magic of food and wine. From the moment you enter the restaurant you feel transported into a world of jovial spirits and fresh ingredients. Chef Richard's style is light and intelligent, with witty presentations and a flair for combining flavors, textures and ingredients.

The decor of Citronelle is a sensual treat all its own, as fresh and bright as the cuisine that graces its tables. Located in the heart of Georgetown at the Latham Hotel, Citronelle features a state of the art glass enclosed exhibition kitchen with Chef's Table, a showcase wine cellar, and private dining rooms for intimate gatherings.

Awarded the James Beard Foundation's 2007 Outstanding Chef, and Outstanding Wine Service, Michel Richard Citronelle exemplifies the art of cuisine.

As an internationally acclaimed chef and restaurateur, Chef Richard is the recipient of the most prestigious culinary honors. His charm has adorned the covers of Gourmet, The Washington Post Magazine, and Washingtonian, and his creativity featured in such publications as Food & Wine, Food Arts, and Bon Appétit, among others.

Chocolate Bar

Total Time: 6 hours including 4 ½ hours of refrigeration

Ingredients:

Bottom Layer

2/3 cup creamy peanut butter

2 Tbsp peanut oil

7 oz milk chocolate melted, and at body temperature

1¼ cups crushed cornflakes

Top Layer:

1 ¼ cups heavy cream

5 oz 60% semisweet chocolate, melted and at body temperature

Hazlenut Sauce (makes ¾ cup)

½ cup granulated sugar

1 Tbsp water

½ cup heavy cream

½ cup whole milk

½ cup (about 2oz) roasted hazelnuts, skins removed (see note)

Unsweetened cocoa powder

1 pint raspberries

Hint: I use organic cornflakes for this recipe because they taste better than ordinary cornflakes. Buy hazelnut with the skins already removed if you can.

Directions:

Line an 8 inch square pan with plastic wrap, letting it overhang on all sides

For the bottom layer, place the peanut butter and oil in the bowl of a stand mixer fitted with the whisk attachment.

Whip on medium to medium-high speed until thoroughly combined and light in color 2 to 3 minutes, stopping to scrape down the sides as necessary.

Reduce the speed to low, add the chocolate, and mix for a minute, or until thoroughly combined.

Remove the bowl from the mixer and stir in the cornflakes.

Pour into the prepared pan.

Using a small offset spatula, spread the mixture into an even layer, being sure to reach into the corners. Cover with plastic wrap and refrigerate until firm, about 30 minutes.

For the top layer, in a bowl of a stand mixer, whip the cream until soft peaks form.

Place the chocolate in a medium to large bowl.

Working fairly quickly - fold half of the whipped cream into the chocolate.

Fold in remaining cream.

Pour the mixture over the bottom layer and spread into an even layer, being sure to reach into the corners. Bang the bottom of the pan against the work surface to eliminate any air bubbles in the top layer.

Cover with plastic wrap and refrigerate until the top layer is set, at least 4 hours. (At this point, the dessert can be refrigerated for up to 3 days)

For the hazelnut sauce, stir the sugar and water together in a medium heavy saucepan over a medium-high heat just to moisten the sugar, and then bring to a boil.

Reduce the heat to a simmer, and cook, without stirring, for about 5 minutes, or until the caramel is light amber. If any sugar crystals cling to the sides of the pan as the caramel cooks, brush them down with a damp pastry brush.

Meanwhile, combine the cream and milk in a small saucepan and heat over medium heat until warm (warming the liquid will help to keep the sugar from hardening when the liquid is added).

Set aside in a warm spot.

When the caramel is light amber, remove the pan from the heat and stir in the hazelnuts, coating them in the caramel.

Return the pan to the heat, add the cream mixture, and bring to a boil.

Reduce the heat and simmer, stirring constantly, for 3 to 4 minutes. The nuts should be thoroughly coated and the caramel liquefied, without any solid pieces. Transfer to a large food processor or blender (be careful, the mixture will be hot).

Cover the top of the feed tube with a towel and process until the nuts are finely ground. Strain through a fine-mesh strainer into a bowl. (The sauce can also be refrigerated, covered, for 3 days).

One hour before serving, remove the pan from the refrigerator. Using the plastic overhang, remove the block from the pan and place on the work surface. Peel off the plastic.

It is best to cut the bars with a warm large knife. Have a deep container of hot water nearby; dip the knife into the water, and dry with a kitchen towel before each cut.

Cut into sixteen 4-by-1-inch bars.

Using a tea strainer, or a fine-mesh sieve, dust the tops of the bars with cocoa powder; brush gently so the cocoa fills in any small holes. Let the cocoa sink in for a minute, then dust a second time for a smooth finish.

Arrange 4 bars on each serving plate. Spoon the sauce around the bars, and garnish with the raspberries.

NOTE: to roast raw un-skinned hazelnuts, preheat oven to 325° F.

Spread the hazelnuts on a baking sheet and toss with ½ to 1 teaspoon of confectioners' sugar, just enough to coat the nuts. Roast for about 5 minutes, then shake the tray to turn the nuts. Continue to roast another 7-8 minutes, or until the nuts are golden and the skins begin to pull away from the nuts. Place about half the nuts in a coarse strainer and rub them against the strainer to remove the skin. Repeat with the remaining nuts.

Recipe makes 4 servings. All values are per serving. **Calories: 1213**, Protein: 22 g, Total Fat: 93 g, Saturated Fat: 40 g

Dante & Luigi's

Corona di ferro

Dante & Luigi's
Corona di ferro

Philadelphia, Pennsylvania

Contributed By: Connie LaRussa

Restaurant Anecdotes

In 1899 "Dante & Luigi's - corona di ferro, Philadelphia's oldest Italian restaurant opened its doors.

It became not only a landmark Philadelphia restaurant, but also a final destination for immigrants entering our city.

Unable to speak our language, they arrived at the docks with the name of the restaurant pinned to their lapels, to be brought here hoping to find lodging on the upper floors of the restaurant, and work in the Italian market area.

Today, 110 years later, with our rich history, the tradition of fine Italian food continues to delight new generations of patrons. The delicious Italian cuisine, excellent service, and "Olde World" charm of our 160 year old Towne House, make this a delightful experience and a "Must Stop" for all visitors to Philadelphia.

We hope you will join us to mangia, and Enjoy!

Connie & Michael LaRussa

Dante & Luigi's

Homemade Manicotti

Total Time: 40 Minutes

Ingredients for Cheese Filling:

1 ½ lbs Ricotta Cheese

¼ lb. Provolone cheese (diced)

1 egg yolk

Small handful of Parmigiana cheese

¼ cup fresh Basil

Black pepper

Directions for Cheese Filling:

Mix all ingredients together, adding more Parmigiana if mixture is too loose

Ingredients for Crepes:

1 cup Flour

2 Eggs

½ cup Milk

½ cup Water

Directions for Crepes:

Mix together to make a thin batter

Pour a small ladle full of batter into a hot pan and coat bottom

Let brown and turn and brown on the other side

Directions for Assembly:

Fill homemade Crepes (or use store bought crepes or Pasta shells) with cheese mixture

Butter tops and bake in a 350° F oven for approximately 15 minutes or until golden brown

Top with Dante & Luigi's "Sugo di Pasta" (our homemade sauce available in our Restaurant) or your favorite tomato sauce

Mangia and enjoy!!

Recipe makes 4 Servings. All values are per serving (2 manicotti). **Calories: 657**, Protein: 39g Total Fat: 38g, Saturated Fat: 22 g

Hudson's on the bend

The Finest Hill Country Cuisine

Austin, Texas

Contributed By: Jeff Blank

Menu

Appetizers

Wild Game Enchiladas with a Chocolate Almond Mole Sauce
Tamale Cheese Pie with Double Smoked Quail

Entrees

Macadamia Nut Crusted Red Snapper with a Mango Butter Sauce
Duck Breast with Red Chili Glaze
Mr. Pibb's Ribs with Sarsasparilla BBQ Sauce

Side Dishes

Hominy and Green Bean Casserole
Mac N' Cheese

Desserts

Tina Turner Mousse

THE RECIPE ARE EXCERPTED WITH PERMISSION FROM
Fired Up by Jeff Blank with Sara Courington Copyright (c) 2005 Laurentius Press AND
COOKING FEARLESSLY by Jeff Blank, Jay Moore, with Deborah Harter
Copyright (c) 1999 Fearless Press

Wild Game Enchiladas with a Chocolate Almond Mole Sauce

Recipe Anecdotes

Mole (mo-lay) to a Mexican is like a bowl of chili to a Texan or a bowl of gumbo to a Cajun, or for that matter turkey stuffing to a New Englander. Each knows that his family recipe is the best. The actual meaning of the word "mole" is a little unclear. Some say it means "sauce," others that it means "mashed" referring to what you do to most of the ingredients. One enthusiastic eater swears that it means "Mucho Ole!" – now that's a definition hard to argue with.

This chocolate almond mole is a wonderfully rich blend of ingredients. For years moles were reserved for special occasions – fiestas- probably because of the time involved and the lengthy shopping list – but it's a great way to stimulate your taste buds and the economy – some people even claim that mole is an aphrodisiac.

Total Time: The mole sauce will store safely in your refrigerator for two weeks.

Freezing is okay if you must. It also makes a wonderful sauce to top grilled chicken or pork. Cooking time: approximately 55 minutes.

TOOLS: Baking Pan or Cookie Sheet, Tongs, Paper Towels, Large Saucepan, Skillet, Bowl, Knife, Food Processor with S-Blade, Cheese Grater, Spice Grinder

Ingredients:

1 lb wild game or beef and pork mix (can be game birds or even chicken), or any combination of the above.

1 large yellow onion, minced

3 ribs celery, minced

1 large carrot, minced

6 cloves garlic, minced

1or 2 jalapenos, minced – if you want it extra spicy leave the seeds and ribs in

1 Tbsp salt, or more

2 Tbsp ground cumin

16 corn tortillas

¾ lb of Monterey Jack cheese, grated

1 cup peanut or canola oil

Directions for the Filling:

Mince onion, carrots, garlic, and jalapeno in a processor with an S-blade. The food processor bowl should b e about ½ full, which is why we always buy the one with the biggest food bowl. Rough chop veggies first; make sure you have a sharp blade. Never overload your food processor

Hand-chop the celery because it gets stringy if chopped in the processor

Grind or mince the meat with a sharp knife or food processor S-blade

Pre-heat a large skillet or saucepan over medium-high heat

Brown meat until most of the fat is rendered off

Add veggies and spices

Simmer 20 minutes and set aside to cool

Directions for the Tortillas:

In a large skillet, heat peanut or canola oil over medium-high heat until it shimmers- 325 – 350° F fry temperature. It's good to have paper towels handy to suck up extra oil.

Using tongs, dip the corn tortillas in the hot oil for 3-4 seconds each and lay them out on the paper towels to drain. If you were in Mexico these would be fried in animal fat – tasty si, healthy no.

Lay out tortillas on the countertop and put about 1 oz of meat and ½ oz. of cheese on each.

Roll them up. Rolling works best while they are still warm from the oil bath.

Place them in a baking pan or casserole, top with sauce, and heat in a 350° F oven for 15 minutes.

Sprinkle with cheese and heat 2 more minutes, and then serve.

Ingredients for the Sauce:

1 cup celery

½ cup carrot

½ cup yellow onion

6 cloves garlic

2 jalapenos, seeds and all

½ cup olive oil

2 Tbsp Mexican oregano (regular will work)

½ cup chili powder

½ cup ancho chili, pureed (rehydrate in water/spin down in blender)

½ cup tomato paste

¼ cup cumin

1 cup almonds, sliced

½ cup sesame seeds

5 cups good chicken stock

½ cup Worcestershire sauce

½ cup brown sugar

8 oz dark semi-sweet chocolate

2 bunches cilantro-leaves only, chopped

2 tsp salt, or to taste

Directions for the Sauté:

Toast ½ cup sesame seeds in a dry skillet until lightly browned. Set aside to cool. Toast almonds the same way. Grind separately in spice grinder.

Mince celery finely by hand before adding to carrots, onions, garlic, and jalapeno in the food processor. Puree until all are mashed together.

Sauté vegetables in very hot olive oil until caramelization just begins.

Add oregano, chili powder, ancho pepper, tomato paste, cumin, almonds, sesame seeds and sauté 8-10 minutes.

In a large saucepan, bring chicken stock, Worcestershire sauce, and brown sugar to a boil.

Add sautéed ingredients and simmer for 10 minutes.

Add chopped cilantro and chopped chocolate.

Remove from heat and stir until chocolate melts into the sauce.

Correct seasoning with salt.

Note: When reheating sauce, bring to a simmer (180° F)

Recipe makes 8 servings. All values are per serving. **Calories: 1014**, Protein: 31 g, Total Fat: 70, Saturated Fat: 22 g

Tamale Cheese Pie with Double Smoked Quail

Recipe Anecdotes

Chef Jeff, Big Homey, Chief Jolly, Butter Boy and Cheese Head are all names that Jeff will answer to! There is an accompanying story for each label. Sometimes he has to pinch himself to see if his life has been a dream.

One day in 1995ish, as a spokesperson for the Dairy Council, he found himself executing the Tamale Cheese Pie with Double-Smoked Quail Topped with Chipotle Mexican Crème in front of 500 of the finest women of the Junior League in Minnesota. "Somebody wake me up. All of my dreams have been fulfilled," he said.

Total Time: Always best when served fresh and eaten immediately, but we all have re-heated quiche in the microwave; cooking time: 50 minutes. Mexican . Crème does require overnight

Variations: Use smoked tenderloin or duck breast, or, as we have learned, you can put anything in a quiche. If you add bacon, you have Quiche Lorraine

Tools: 9" pie tin, Box grater, Food processor, Whisk, Plastic wrap

Ingredients for Crust:

1 cup masa (Maseca® or Quaker Oat brand)

2 Tbsp butter, cubed and cold

1 Tbsp chili powder (we always prefer a blend of ancho, chipotle, and New Mexico chili powders)

1 tsp salt

1 cup water

Directions for Crust:

Mix the chili powder, masa, and salt.

Cut cold butter into masa with a fork or pulse in a food processor until the old butter is pea size.

Add the water and blend until dough is formed

Press into a 9" pie tin and bake for 15 minutes at 325° F. (just like prebaking pie crust)

Set aside to cool

Ingredients for Filling

½ cup jalapeno Jack cheese, grated

½ cup cheddar cheese, grated

1 cup red onion, ¼" diced

1 Tbsp garlic, minced

1 poblano pepper, ¼" diced

2 Tbsp chili powder mix

4 eggs

1 cup heavy cream

2 smoked quail, ¼" diced (approximately 8 ounces)

1 ½ tsp salt

Directions for the Filling:

Whisk heavy cream and eggs together

Add garlic, onion, pepper, quail, chili powder and salt to egg mix

Sprinkle cheese into tamale shell

Pour egg mixture into the tamale shell

Bake for 50 minutes at 350° F

Let the pie rest 10 minutes before serving.

Ingredients for the Chili powder Mix:

Equal parts:

Ancho chili powder

Chipotle chili powder

New Mexico chili powder

San Antonion chili powder

Upscale or ethnic markets have the best selection of chili powders. We advise buying as many as possible and making your own custom blend. Just remember some are quite hot. Jalapeno and chipotle powders pack a wallop.

Ingredients for Mexican Crème:

½ cup ancho puree (6 ancho chilies, seeded; 2 cups warm water)

Soak the ancho chilies in water for 30 minutes or until soft

Puree in blender. To encourage the puree add a little of the chilies water

2 cups heavy cream

½ cup buttermilk (active buttermilk, not ultra-pasteurized buttermilk*)

Directions for Mexican crème

Mix the heavy cream and buttermilk together

Let the mixture sit out overnight in a glass (nonreactive) bowl covered with Saran Wrap. This is much like making yogurt

Mix in ancho puree

Dollop on pie

*Active buttermilk is sold in the dairy section as "buttermilk for baking." Modern dairies kill the bacteria in buttermilk. Bacteria are a must for most baking. With this active buttermilk, the French create a topping called crème fraiche, Mexicans call it Mexican crème.

Recipe makes 6 servings. All values are per serving. **Calories: 749**, Protein: 24 g, Total Fat: 64 g, Saturated Fat: 37 g

Macadamia Nut Crusted Red Snapper with a Mango Butter Sauce

Recipe Anecdotes

We have a new obsession with macadamia nuts and oil. It is due to the fact that we love the richness and flavor of the nuts. They are monounsaturated and are as healthy if not more so, than extra virgin olive oils. According to the every reliable source of People Magazine, the stars eat 2 tablespoons of macadamia nut oil a day to boost their metabolism. They are very heart healthy! What a bonus to find something this rich and tasty that is also good for your heart. If you have trouble finding the macadamia nut oil, go to www.macnutoil.com. It is a great item to keep on hand in your pantry.

Total Time: Sauce can be prepared 1 hour in advance. Breading can be made days in advance. Fish can be breaded the morning of your dinner.

Variations: Orange roughy, red fish, halibut. Use the freshest lightest flaky fish available. It is important that the filets not be more than ¾" thick.

Timing: Sauce can be prepared 1 hour in advance. Breading can be made days in advance. Fish can be breaded the morning of your dinner.

Ingredients for Mango Butter Sauce:

2 cups dry white wine, sauvignon blanc or chenin blanc

1 large shallot, rough chopped

4 cloves garlic, crushed

4 limes, juiced and zested

½ cup honey

½ cup heavy cream

3 mangos, pitted and peeled (one of these mangos is ¼" diced and reserved for garnish)

½ tsp sea salt

1 jalapeno pepper

2 sticks butter, cubed at room temperature

Directions for Mango Butter Sauce:

In a medium saucepan, over high heat, reduce the wine to 1/4 cup of amber liquid

Add the shallot, garlic, zest, lime juice, honey, cream, mangos, sea salt, and jalapeno pepper. Simmer for 5 minutes over medium heat

Pour the simmering mixture from the saucepan into a blender. Be certain to vent the steam and then blend on high.

Add the butter, a couple of chunks at a time until all of the butter has been added.

Adjust the salt level and store in a thermal pitcher until serving.

Ingredients for Macadamia Herb Crusted Red Snapper

6 Filets of red snapper, skinless and boneless (6 to 7 ounces each)

4 cups macadamia nuts

2 cups panko bread crumbs

3 Tbsp Chinese Five-Spice mix

1½ Tbsp sea salt

Egg wash (3 eggs and 1 cup milk)

2 cups all-purpose flour

½ cup macadamia nut oil

Directions for Macadamia Herb Crusted Red Snapper:

Put macadamia nuts in a food processor with the S-blade and pulse until the nuts are corn kernel size. Some will be smaller

Add the panko bread crumbs, Chinese Five-Spice mix and salt to the food processor.

Pulse until blended. Do not over blend. You want some texture

Set up your breading station *

Bread the snapper filets using the standard breading procedure.

Heat a large sauté pan on medium high heat with the macadamia nut oil to 350° F.

This temperature is reached just before the oil begins smoking. Hint: A small piece of lettuce will pop when it is dropped in the oil.

Cook 2 filets at a time for about 4 minutes on each side until a rich golden brown.

Place the cooked filet on a cookie sheet in a warm oven (200° F) while you finish cooking the snapper

Assembly

Place the cooked snapper filets on the dinner plate.

Top with 3 ounces of sauce

Garnish with diced mango and peppers

*Standard Breading Procedure

You will need 3 casserole dishes or baking pans

Put 2 cups of all-purpose flour in one baking pan

Make your egg wash with 3 eggs and 1 cup of milk whisked together and put the mixture in the second baking pan.

The third container will hold the breading

Bread one piece of snapper at a time. Begin by dragging the snapper through the flour.

Shake off the excess flour

Dip the snapper into the egg wash until all of the flour is wet.

Press the snapper into the breading lightly with your hand.

Set the snapper on a cookie sheet and continue until all the snappers are coated. Be certain to spread the snapper filets evenly on the cookie sheet. Do not stack them. Unlike some of our breading recipes, this one can be done several hours in advance.

Refrigerate until cooking time.

Recipe makes 6 servings. All values are per serving. **Calories: 1382**, Protein: 45 g, Total Fat: 123 g, Saturated Fat: 39 g

Duck Breast with Red Chili Glaze

Recipe Anecdotes

Glaze and amaze! A glaze is a light brushed-on-sauce. We feel that the best glazes are ones that have both a savory and a sweet side. In this recipe the smoke from the grill combines with the salty soy, the tart vinegar, and the sweet brown sugar for an amazing taste treat.

You can now buy ready-to-cook duck breast at butcher counters in good grocery stores. This is much easier than trying to de-bone the whole bird. All farm-raised duck has a layer of fat between the skin and the meat. When properly grilled over a hardwood fire the fat will be cooked away and the skin will be crisp.

Total Time: Glaze can easily be made a day or two in advance. Cooking time: approximately 30 minutes

Variations: This glaze is also great with chicken and pork.

Ingredients:

8 Duck Breasts (1 per person)

Red Chili Glaze

Directions for Duck Breast

Score the skin and fat layer of the raw bird with a sharp knife in a crosshatch pattern

Lightly season with salt and pepper

Place the duck breast, skin side down, over a hot charcoal or hardwood fire. Keep a watchful eye as the duck fat will begin to cook out and the fire will flare up. If this happens, move the breast to the side until it dies down. Flame-kissed duck skin will become crispy and delicious

Cook the breast skin-side down for the majority of the grill time- approximately 8 minutes depending on the heat of the fire. Turn breast over and grill the inside for 2 minutes maximum. You'll find that most good restaurants serve duck medium rare to medium, so don't be afraid of a little pinkness on the inside

Slice the duck breast and fan it out on the plate to increase the eye appeal

Serve topped with Red Chili Glaze

Ingredients for Red Chili Glaze

1 cup champagne vinegar

1 to 1 ½ Tbsp red chili flakes (if you like it hot use 1½ to 2 tablespoons flakes; if not, use 1 tablespoon or less)

1 Tbsp garlic, minced

2 Tbsp onions, minced

2 cups light brown sugar, packed

2 Tbsp tomato paste

½ cup soy sauce

1 tsp salt

1 stick sweet butter, cut into 8-10 chunks

Directions for Red Chili Glaze:

Simmer champagne vinegar, chili flakes, garlic and onion in a heavy saucepan until reduced by half

Add brown sugar, tomato paste, soy sauce and salt and bring back to a simmer for 3 minutes

Remove from heat and whisk in butter chunks. This glaze can burn easily so brush it on just prior to serving

Recipe makes 8 servings. All values are per serving. **Calories: 457**, Protein: 25 g, Total Fat: 14 g, Saturated Fat: 7 g

Mr. Pibb's Ribs with Sarsasparilla BBQ Sauce

Recipe Anecdotes

Evolution in the kitchen never stops. In the spirit of Hudson's, we have added layer upon layer of changes to this recipe.

To tell the story of the conception of this recipe, we must first give you the family tree.

In the beginning, there was Jay Moore, former chief of Hudson's. He went to school at the Culinary Institute of America. There he roomed with Jim Fisher. While at Hudson's, Jay hired Becky Barsch. Becky Barsch was introduced to Jim Fisher by Jay Moore. Becky Barsch became Becky Barsch-Fisher.

Out of this union was born the Coco-Cola Baby Back Ribs, a long-standing favorite on the menu at Hudson's on the Bend. We think this recipe was acquired through a little pillow talk in the Fisher house. Apparently, the love of a recipe trumps all loves.

Total Time: BBQ sauce can be made in advance. It has a long shelf life. Marinate ribs 48 hours in advance; cooking time 30 minutes for the sauce.. Slow cook the ribs until tender and falling off the bone

Ingredients for Baby Back Rib Marinade:

4 quarts Mr. Pibb (or Dr. Pepper)

1 cup of hoya santas, minced

¼ cup salt

3 cups dark, dark, dark brown sugar (use a little black strap molasses if you can't get real dark sugar)

3 to 4 racks of babyback pork ribs

Directions for Baby Back Ribs:

Place all ingredients, except the ribs, in a large pot and simmer until the sugar and salt go into solution.
Cool mixture

Submerge the ribs in the marinade and hold in refrigerator for 48 hours. (Extra large Ziploc bags work great.)

Salt the ribs and slow cook over low smoky embers until the ribs are tender and falling off the bone.

Ingredients for Sarsasparilla BBQ Sauce:

¼ cup garlic, minced

¼ cup onion, minced

1 stick butter

¼ cup fresh ginger, minced

2 cups root beer

½ cup hoya santas, minced

¼ cup molasses

¼ cup dark brown sugar

1 cup ketchup

¼ cup Worcestershire sauce

¼ cup lime juice

¼ cup orange juice

2 tsp salt

2 TBSP Tabasco sauce

Directions for Sarsasparilla BBQ Sauce:

Simmer the butter, garlic, and onion in a saucepan until they sweat

Add the other ingredients and simmer for 30 minutes
Serve with the slow cooked ribs

Recipe makes 10 servings. All Values are per serving. **Calories: 1187**, Protein: 74 g, Total Fat: 87 g, Saturated Fat: 34 g

Hominy and Green Bean Casserole

Recipe Anecdotes

Perini Ranch in Buffalo Gap Texas, top 10 in Gourmet Magazine.

In the beginning, Perini Ranch was out in the country and far, far away from the eyes of the Department of Agriculture. Lo and behold, in 2001 the New York Times picked Tom's famous smoked tenderloins as one of the top 10 recommended gifts to ship to loved ones for Christmas. But, as all celebrities can attest, along with fame comes undesirable attention.

Everyone in the country started taking note of Tom's tenders. The USDA called Tom to check on his type of tenderloin and his method of smoking, and informed him of the need for a permit to sell and transport tenders across state lines. The USDA call on a daily basis. Tom answered these daily phone calls in a high-pitched woman's voice "Tom's not here".

Well, Tom discovered that you can run, but, you can't hide from the USDA. He eventually walked the walk through the maze of legal red tape and within several weeks had a license to ship worldwide. Since then he has cooked for Bush and Putin at the Ranch and has even gone to Moscow to smoke his world famous tenderloins.

Tom is famous for his tenderloins. But it was his hominy casserole that got our attention. We stole this little side dish that he serves with the tenderloin. This recipe is a twisted and turned version of Tom Perini's Hominy Casserole. We think our recipe is a wee bit more civilized. With the "change three ingredients" rule, a recipe usually ends up with an abundance of ingredients and flavors. We think this one has acquired some unique complexity in its flavor.

Total Time: Casserole can be prepared earlier in the day, baked 1 hour prior to service: Baking time: 50 minutes

<u>Ingredients</u>:

3 16 ounce cans yellow hominy

1 pound blanched* green beans cut into 1" lengths

1 pound bacon, cooked and drained

1 cup Hatch New Mexico chilies, roasted, peeled, seeded, and ¼" diced

1 cup red onion, ¼" diced

1/3 cup garlic, minced

½ TBSP dark chili powder (ancho)

½ TBSP cumin

½ TBSP sage

½ TBSP oregano

1 TBSP salt

¼ cup brown sugar

1 cup cheddar cheese

1 cup Monterey Jack cheese

2 cups Panko bread crumbs

10 whole eggs (cooked in boiling salted water for 1 minute and then shock in ice water to preserve color and crispness)

Directions:

Preheat oven to 375° F

Drain hominy

Chop cooked bacon into ¼" pieces

Mix hominy, green beans, onion, bacon, garlic, chili powder, Hatch chile, cumin, sage, brown sugar, oregano, and salt in a bowl

Whisk 10 eggs

Pour the whisked eggs into the hominy mixture

Pour into 9" X 12" casserole

Layer cheese on top and cover with Panko bread crumbs

Bake at 375° F for 50 minutes.

Recipe makes 9 servings. All values are per serving. **Calories: 376,** Protein: 18 g, Total Fat: 16 g, Saturated Fat: 7 g.

Mac N' Cheese

Recipe Anecdotes

Immediately after 9/11, everyone was craving comfort food. This one appeared on our menu as a result of Becky's need to comfort the world with her God-given talents. She elevated the lowly Mac n'Cheese to a gourmet level. Though the veal meatloaf with a foie gras center and the buffalo hamburger did not survive on our menu, the Truffled Mac n' Cheese lives on at Hudson's.

Total Time: This can be prepared in advance, refrigerated, and baked at the last minute. Baking time: 25 minutes

Ingredients:

1 pound dried pasta (macaroni, penne, cavatappi)

¼ cup truffle oil

1 quart heavy cream

½ stick of butter

6 TBSP all-purpose flour

Dash cayenne pepper

Salt and pepper to taste

1 cup grated Parmesan

1 cup Boursin® cheese

1 truffle

1 cup bread crumbs

1 TBSP truffle oil

3 TBSP melted butter

2 TBSP fresh herbs (parsley and chives)

Directions:

Cook pasta in a large pot of boiling salted water, until just tender

Cool pasta with ice and then drain in colander

Toss pasta with ¼ cup truffle oil

Melt ½ stick butter in a heavy bottomed saucepan

Stir in flour to make a blonde roux (don't brown)

Add heavy cream and simmer mixture until it thickens

Season with cayenne, salt and pepper

Remove from heat and add pasta and cheeses

Stir to combine

Taste Mixture and adjust salt and pepper if needed

Pour into a buttered oven proof casserole dish

In a bowl, combine bread crumbs, melted butter, 1 tablespoon of truffle oil, and herbs

Pour bread crumbs over the pasta cheese mixture

Bake until golden brown at 400° to 425° F for approximately 25 minutes

Garnish with truffle slices (optional)

This can be prepared in advance, refrigerated and baked at the last minute

Garnish: Truffle slices or more grated cheese

Recipe makes 10 servings. All values are per serving. **Calories: 741**, Protein: 13 g, Total Fat: 56 g, Saturated Fat: 29 g.

Tina Turner Mousse

Recipe Anecdotes

Making a dessert in honor of an entertainer is as old as Escoffier. He created Peach Melba in 1899 as a tribute to Madame Nellie Melba, the great diva, commemorating the swan from the first act of Logengrin. An Australian dessert is named for the Russian ballerina, Anna Pavlova, a confection of meringue, whipped cream, passion fruit, kiwi and pineapple.

This dessert is dedicated to a contemporary diva, Tina Turner, a performer known for her unforgettable voice and great legs. "Legs" is also the term used to describe streams of wine that cling and then slide down the inside of a glass when wine is swirled. In this dish it is swirling chocolate making a tempting presentation, a fitting tribute, and a great tasting dessert.

The best way to deal with temptation is to give into it.

Total Time: Best if made no earlier than the morning of your dinner party. Preparation time approximately two and a half hours

Variation: If you don't have Chambord®, try Grand Marnier®, Framboise, or Tuaca®

Ingredients for Chambord Mousse:

1 cup Chambord® liqueur

4 oz semi-sweet chocolate

2 cups heavy cream

½ cup granulated sugar

1 pint raspberries

Directions for Chambord Mousse:

In a small saucepan, simmer liqueur until reduced to ¼ cup, and cool

Melt chocolate in a double boiler or in a bowl over simmering water. Stir until smooth and transfer into stainless bowl. Hold at room temperature

Whip the heavy cream and sugar in a well-chilled bowl with an electric mixer. As the cream begins to form soft peaks, add the Chambord syrup in a slow steady stream. Stop mixing at medium-firm peaks.

Take 1 cup of the Chambord whipped cream and fold it into the chocolate. Vigorously whisk the two together until well blended. This will keep the chocolate from seizing up when blending with cold whipped cream mixture

Add the chocolate cream mixture to the remaining whipped cream and gently fold together until smooth

Chill for two hours

Ingredients for Chocolate Fudge:

2 cups cream

½ stick butter

1 cup brown sugar

1 cup granulated sugar

¼ tsp salt

2 cups Dutch cocoa, sifted

Directions for Chocolate Fudge and Preparation:

In a saucepan, combine heavy cream and butter. Bring to a boil

Add brown and granulated sugars and salt

Bring back to a boil and stir, making sure all the sugar is dissolved

Remove from the heat and whisk in cocoa, ½ cup at a time.

Whisk vigorously until all cocoa has been added. Hold at warm room temperature, or near warm stove

Make "legs of fudge" in a wine glass or tall parfait

Load a pastry bag with chilled mousse and fill fudged wine glass ½ full

Garnish with raspberries

Recipe makes 6 servings. All values are per serving. **Calories: 1160**, Protein: 8 g, Total Fat: 79 g, Saturated Fat: 48 g

IBIZA
RESTAURANT

New Haven, Connecticut

Contributed By: Manuel Romero

Restaurant Anecdotes

IBIZA is a very special Spanish restaurant, where the traditional and the modern fuse in a coherent way. While traditional flavors are kept, we use new techniques, reflecting the new culinary revolution and, where flavors and aromas play, a very important role in the creation of our dishes.

About the Chef

Manuel Romero born in La Coruna, Spain, and came to the USA, New York, at the age of 14 in the year of 1988. After finishing High School, he went to the New York Technical College of Brooklyn to study Hospitality Management. After one year of studies in that field, he specialized in the culinary arts.

His first experience in the area of restaurants was in 1999 as an assistant of Chef Luis Bollo in Meigas restaurant located in New York City. Due to his dedication and love for the good cuisine he got the position of sous chef at the same restaurant.

He also worked at the Hyatt Hotel in New York City and Meson Galicia restaurant located in Norwalk, Connecticut. In 2001, after several months in Spain improving his culinary skills, he was hired as a sous chef in Café Pika Tapas (New Haven, CT). One year later changed its name and the concept of the cuisine, becoming Ibiza restaurant. As an Executive Chef, he participated in several culinary events as: Flavors of CT, Mohegan Sun Casino, Foxwoods Food and Wine Festival, as well as Connecticut television shows, magazines and cookbooks and local events.

Seared Salmon with Pistachio Vinaigrette and Catalan Style Spinach

Total Time: 45 minutes

Ingredients:

4 Salmon fillets (7 ounce each)

4 TBSP vegetable oil

1 pound baby spinach

2 ounces pine nuts

3 ounces raisins

3 TBSP sherry vinegar

7 TBSP extra virgin olive oil

1.5 ounce crushed roasted pistachios

6 ounces diced tomatoes

1 TBSP lemon juice

Salt and pepper

Directions for vinaigrette:

Stir together vinegar, 7 tablespoons extra virgin olive oil and lemon juice in a small bowl

Add the crushed pistachios and tomatoes.

Taste for salt and pepper

Directions for salmon:

Heat vegetable oil in a nonstick skillet.

Increase heat to high

Add the salmon and sear until well brown

Turn fish over and sear until just cooked through

Directions for Spinach:

Heat 3 tablespoons olive oil in a pan over moderate heat until hot but not smoking

Add the pine nuts and raisins and cook stirring until pine nuts are golden

Add spinach by the handful, stirring, and cook until wilted and tender for about four minutes

Season with salt

Transfer the salmon to plates and add the vinaigrette over.

Place the spinach next to it

Recipe makes 4 servings. All calories are per serving. **Calories: 1065**, Protein: 55g, Total Fat: 78g, Saturated Fat: 13g

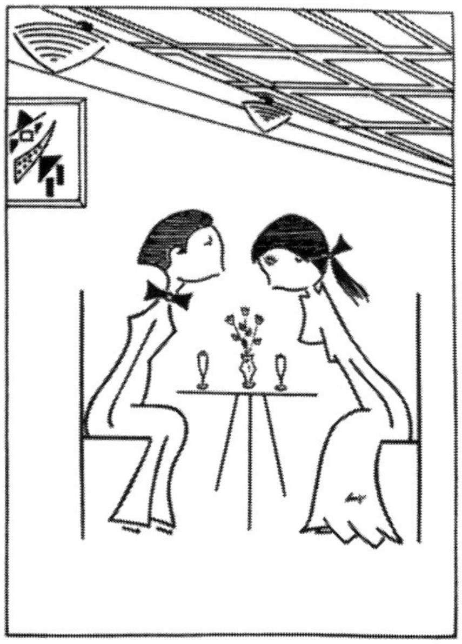

Jean-Louis

Today, tomorrow and since 1985

Greenwich, Connecticut

Contributed By: Master Chef of France, Jean-Louis Gerin

Restaurant Anecdotes

Since opening in 1985, restaurant JEAN-LOUIS has earned a reputation as perhaps the finest restaurant in Connecticut, and one of the best in the United States. Recognized by Wine Spectator for more than seventeen years for its excellent wine list, and consistently given top ratings by Zagat and newspapers from the New York Times to the San Diego Chronicle, restaurant JEAN-LOUIS is simultaneously noted for its fine cuisine and utter lack of pretense. Most recently, Chef Jean-Louis Gerin was given his food "Oscar" when announced as the Best Chef, Northeast at the 2006 James Beard Awards.

"Over the past 20 years, my cuisine has matured into a unique style of Modern French. This richly flavored cuisine is complex yet light, and the cooking method uses elaborate techniques and the latest technologies with a constant respect for my classical training."
Jean-Louis Gerin

Beef Cheeks slowly Braised in Red Wine with Onion Compote and Foie Gras

Total Time: 3 to 5 Hours

Ingredients:

1 750-milliliter bottle red wine

2 sprigs thyme

2 beef cheeks, or 1 2-pound piece beef brisket (about 1"thick), with some of fat cap left untrimmed

4 Tbsp olive oil

1-3 Tbsp olive oil

1-3 Tbsp butter

1 Tbsp minced garlic

1 bay leaf

1 cup veal stock (see note)

3 medium yellow onions, peeled, halved, and thinly sliced (to make about 4 cups sliced onions)

4 slices fresh foie gras (see note)

Directions:

Preheat oven to 325° F

Bring wine and thyme to a boil in a medium saucepan set over high heat

Boil until reduced by half (to about 1 ½ cups), about 15 minutes, then set aside

Pat beef cheeks or brisket dry with paper towel, then season with salt and pepper on flesh (not fatty) side

Heat 1 tablespoon of the olive oil with 1 tablespoon butter in a medium, heavy-bottomed pot set over medium-high heat.

Brown meat well all over, starting with fatty side down and finishing with fatty side up, about 5 minutes per side

Without removing meat from the pot, pour off and discard fat

Return pot to medium-high heat and add the reduced red wine, garlic, and bay leaf.

When liquid boils, add the veal stock.

Bring to a boil, then transfer pot to the oven

Cook uncovered for half an hour, then cover and continue cooking until meat is extremely tender, 2 ½ - 3 hours

Caramelize the onions: Heat remaining 3 tablespoons olive oil in a large sauté pan set over medium heat.

Add the sliced onion and cook, stirring occasionally, until deep brown in color, 30-45 minutes. If onions start to dry out, add a knob or two of butter and stir more frequently.

To serve, slice each beef cheeks or brisket.

Layer slices of meat with caramelized onion and foie gras in each of four bowls. Adjust seasoning of the cooking sauce to taste with salt and pepper, and drizzle over the foie gras.

NOTE: At the restaurant, we of course use our rich homemade veal stock! However, if you don't make your own, this recipe works well with the "Perfect Additions' brand of frozen veal stock; merely defrost the stock and use it full strength (do not dilute, despite what it may say on the container). Slices of fresh foie gras can be found at most gourmet markets – use as much or as little as desired!

Recipe makes 4 Servings. All values are per serving. **Calories: 1157** Protein: 53 g, Total Fat: 103 g, Saturated Fat: 37 g

Atlanta, Georgia

Contributed By: Chef Cyrille Holota

Restaurant Anecdotes

JOËL BRASSERIE is a chic yet relaxed French restaurant founded on blending contemporary style with rustic flavors. Responsible for one of Atlanta's most acclaimed dining experiences, Chef Cyrille Holota guides the kitchen as executive chef and brings his full-flavored brasserie concept to the menu. The Brasserie offers two gorgeous private rooms, a breath taking 3,000 sq. ft. kitchen, and a wine cellar which houses over 3,000 bottles.

Menu Selections

Pommes Maxime (Thin Potato Crisps)
Croque Monsieur

Pommes Maxime (Thin Potato Crisps)

Total Time: 30-35 minutes

Ingredients:

2 lbs Potatoes

Butter

Parchment paper

Directions:

Peel and wash the potatoes

Slice the potatoes very fine (Slicer #15)

Cut them into the desired shape

Lay the potato shapes on some buttered parchment paper, laid on a tray. Top with another sheet of parchment paper and cover with another tray.

Cook in the oven at 250°F for about 16 minutes (check on the potatoes regularly).

Recipe makes 5 Servings. All values are per serving. **Calories:158,** Protein:3.9 g, Total Fat:1.76 g, Saturated Fat: 0.9 g

Croque Monsieur

Total Time : 20 minutes

Ingredients:

Fresh Country bread 1 loaf

White ham 8 slices

Gruyere cheese (Swiss) 8 oz

Butter 3 oz

Flour 3 oz

Nutmeg 1 pinch

Salt 1 pinch

Pepper 1 pinch

Milk 16 oz

Directions for Béchamel Sauce:

Melt the butter and add the flour to it.

Cook slightly and add in the milk. The mix will become thicker, stir well.

Add the salt, pepper, nutmeg and continue to cook for 4-5 minutes. (If mix is too thick, add milk)

Directions:

Slice and toast the bread

Spread some Béchamel sauce on a slice of bread, lay 2 slices of ham, the Swiss cheese and finally the Béchamel sauce

Close the sandwich

On top of the sandwich, spread some more Béchamel sauce and place in a 350°F oven for 10 minutes

Recipe makes 4 sandwiches. All values are per serving. **Calories: 785**, Protein: 41 g, Total Fat: 42 g, Saturated Fat: 22 g

La Bonne Auberge

Classic French Cuisine
since 1972

New Hope, Pennsylvania

Contributed By: Rozanne Caronello

Restaurant Anecdotes

La Bonne Auberge is a charming 250 years old farm house renowned for its exquisite food in elegant surroundings. Highly rated by Zagat, AAA, Wine Spectator, and Dirona. It has maintained its excellence for 37 years.

Potage Parmentier Leek and Potato Soup

Total Time: 1 hour

Ingredients:

3 large leeks (white part only – soak and clean carefully)

1 large Spanish onion

6 large potatoes

¼ lb butter

Heavy cream (1 cup per gallon of water – see directions below)

Directions:

Slice onions and leeks finely

Peel and cut potatoes into small pieces – keep on side

Cook onions and leeks in butter in a large saucepan until the vegetables have rendered their juices without changing color

Add 1 gallon of water and bring to a boil

Add potatoes and cook for approximately 25-30 minutes

Grind ingredients in a Cuisinart and season accordingly. This mixture can be refrigerated and small portions can be used as needed

For serving, add cream to the required amount and serve hot or cold.

Garnish with freshly chopped chives.

Recipe makes 6-8 servings. All values are per serving. **Calories: 431**, Protein: 6g, Total Fat: 26 g, Saturated Fat: 16 g

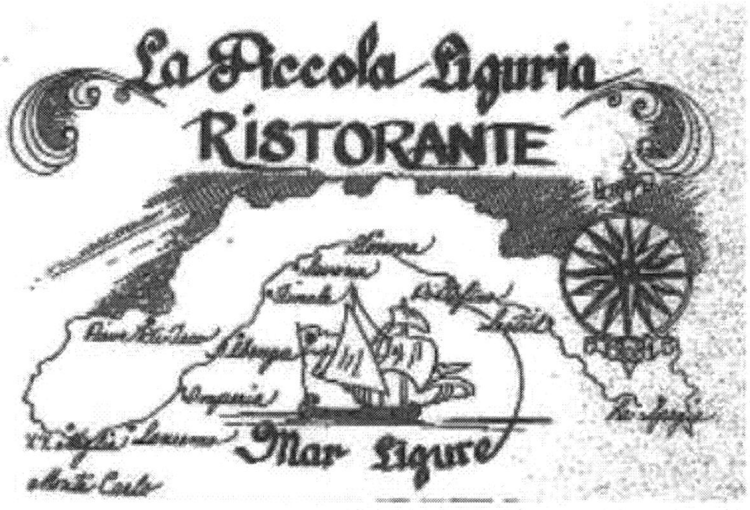

Port Washington, NY

Contributed By: Victor Raimondo

Restaurant Anecdotes

It's "worth a trip from anywhere on the Island" to this tiny Port Washington destination for the "creative", "amazing", "authentic Northern Italian cuisine" that's served "with great panache" by an "impressive" staff that can recite a list of "seemingly hundreds of wonderful specials"; though the "décor won't win any awards", the atmosphere's "warm", and for many connoisseurs "it doesn't get any better than this."

Bow Tie Pasta a la Liguria

Total Time: 30 minutes includes cooking the pasta

Ingredients:

8 ounces Farfalle

1 cup diced baby string beans

1 cup diced potato

Directions for Farfalle:

Cook Farfalle, Baby String Beans and Diced Potato separately

Put aside

Ingredients for Pesto Sauce:

A handful of Basil Leaves

1 garlic Clove

A handful of Pignoli Nuts

A pinch of Salt

Directions for Pesto Sauce:

Prepare the Pesto ingredients in a food processor using a low speed

Add ½ tsp Extra Virgin Olive Oil

Directions for Preparation:

Place the following ingredients together: pasta, string beans, diced potato and add a touch of butter and blend together

Add pesto sauce

Finish with Parmesan cheese

Recipe makes 4 servings. All values are per serving. **Calories: 479**, Protein: 21 g, Total Fat: 19 g, Saturated Fat: 4 g

Nora

Washington, DC

Contributed By: Nora Pouillon

Restaurant Anecdotes

Restaurant NORA, the first USDA certified organic restaurant in the country, has always stood for sustainable living, healthy food and a concern for the environment. Nora Pouillon, the chef and owner of NORA, has supported the organic food movement through her work at the restaurant since its inception thirty years ago and has become an institution in Washington, D.C. The menu reflects Nora's passion for using the finest ingredients the seasons can offer and showcases Nora's passion for healthy seasonal organic food.

Menu

Caesar Salad with Farm Fresh Eggs
Garlic Croutons & Parmesan
Chicken Breast with Goat Cheese & Walnut Stuffing
Potato Gratin
Fudgy Brownies

Caesar Salad with Farm Fresh Eggs
Garlic Croutons & Parmesan

Total Time: 30 minutes if you cook the eggs and make the croutons from scratch

*Please buy organic ingredients whenever available.

Ingredients for Salad:

4 heads baby romaine lettuce (or 1 large head), trimmed, washed, dried and torn into bite-size pieces

3 eggs, hard-boiled and quartered

4 to 6oz wedge of Parmesan cheese

Caesar Dressing:

2 tsp minced garlic

2 anchovy filets

1 Tbsp Worcestershire sauce

2 tsp Dijon mustard

2 Tbsp grated Parmesan cheese

¼ cup water

1 Tbsp lemon juice

Freshly ground black pepper

½ cup olive oil

Directions:

Put all the ingredients except the olive oil in a blender and blend until smooth.

With blender running, slowly add the oil in a thin stream until the dressing is emulsified and creamy. If too thick, dilute with water.

Ingredients for Garlic Croutons:

1 tsp minced garlic

1 Tbsp olive oil or as needed

Sea salt and freshly ground black pepper

⅓ loaf French or Italian country bread, cut into ½ inch cubes (about 30 cubes)

Directions:

Preheat oven to 425° F

Mix garlic, olive oil, salt and pepper in a medium bowl

Add the bread cubes and toss to coat

Spread the cubes on a baking sheet and bake for 12 to 15 minutes in 425° F oven

Stir once or twice so that the cubes are lightly browned and crispy

Remove from oven and cool

Assembly:

Toss the romaine with the Caesar dressing and divide on 4 plates

Add 3 egg quarters to each plate and sprinkle salad with croutons

Shave thin slices of Parmesan on each salad to garnish

Recipe makes 4 servings. All values are per serving. **Calories: 526**, Protein: 21 g, Total Fat: 46 g, Saturated Fat: 12 g

Chicken Breast with Goat Cheese & Walnut Stuffing

Total Time: 30 minutes with the cooking time for the stuffing, etc.

* Please buy organic ingredients whenever available.

Ingredients:

4 boneless chicken breasts

Salt and pepper for seasoning

1 Tbsp olive oil + 1 Tbsp butter

Stuffing:

2 oz spinach, cleaned

2 Tbsp shallots, minced

1 Tbsp garlic, minced

2 Tbsp olive oil

Salt & pepper to taste

Pinch of mace

4 oz. goat cheese or fromage blanc

2 oz walnuts, toasted & roughly chopped

Directions:

Sauté spinach with shallots and garlic in olive oil.

Season with salt, pepper, and mace.

Cool

Mix with goat cheese and walnuts

Heat oven to 400° F

Make a slit horizontally in chicken breast and insert ¼ of the stuffing.

Close and fold the excess skin over

Season the chicken breast with salt and pepper

Heat oil and butter in a skillet and brown skin side down for 4-5 minutes.

Turn chicken breast over and finish cooking in oven for another 10-12 minutes or until cooked through

Recipe makes: 4 servings. All values are per serving. **Calories: 429**, Protein: 34g, Total Fat: 31g, Saturated Fat: 9g

Potato Gratin

Total Time: For the Potato Gratin, preparation time is 15 – 20 minutes. Nora suggests slicing the potatoes with a mandolin to shorten the prep time. Cooking time takes 1 -1 ½ hours.

*Please buy organic ingredients whenever available.

Ingredients:

2 lb Russet potatoes (5 or more) peeled and sliced into ¼" thick rounds

2 Tbsp butter

1 clove garlic, finely minced

1 cup cream

½ tsp salt

¼ tsp black pepper, freshly ground

1/8 tsp teaspoon nutmeg (optional)

Directions:

Preheat oven to 350° F

Butter a shallow, preferable earthenware gratin dish

Layer the potato slices into the dish, seasoning with salt, pepper, nutmeg and garlic in between the layers

Pour cream over the potatoes – it should come ¾ way up the gratin dish.

Dot with small pieces of butter and bake for 1 – 1 ½ hours until the potatoes are soft and the top is browned and crispy.

Recipe makes 4 servings. All values are per serving. **Calories: 440**, Protein: 6 g, Total Fat: 28 g, Saturated Fat: 17 g

Fudgy Brownies

Total Time: 15 minutes to prepare plus baking time

Please buy organic ingredients whenever available.

<u>Ingredients</u>:

8 oz butter (2 sticks)

8 oz chocolate

4 eggs

½ tsp salt

1 cup sugar

1 cup dark brown sugar

2 tsp vanilla essence

1 cup flour

Chocolate chips (white and dark)

<u>Directions</u>:

Preheat oven to 240° F

Melt butter and chocolate over low heat

Combine eggs, salt, sugars and vanilla essence and whisk with beaters until thick.

Fold in melted butter and chocolate; then gently fold in flour.

Pour into a buttered and flowered 11 x 17 inch jellyroll pan or a parchment lined pan

Sprinkle chocolate chips over the surface

Bake for about 25 to 30 minutes. DO NOT OVERCOOK

Cool in the pan and cut into 2 inch squares

Serve with whipped cream and/or ice cream.

Recipe makes 40 2x2 brownies. All values are per serving. **<u>Calories: 121</u>**, Protein: 1g, Total Fat: 7g, Saturated Fat: 4g

Serving with ¼ cup premium ice cream **<u>adds 92 calories</u>**, 1g protein, 6g total fat and 4g saturated fat

Serving with ¼ cup whipped cream **<u>adds 104 calories</u>**, 0 g protein, 11g total fat and 7g saturated fat

AT FOUR SEASONS HOTEL ATLANTA

Atlanta, Georgia

Contributed By: Robert Gerstenecker

Restaurant Anecdotes

Park 75 Restaurant at Four Seasons Hotel Atlanta is a lively place for dinner, drinks and laughter with friends and family.

Based on the concept of "Southern Steak Redefined"- Park 75's menu incorporates mostly protein-fused with local ingredients, including those grown in Executive Chef Robert Gerstenecker's garden on the hotel's rooftop.

Park 75 is one of only two Mobil Four-Star restaurants in Georgia. The restaurant is located inside Four Seasons Hotel Atlanta at 75 14th Street.

Crab Mac-n-Cheese

Total Time: 30 Minutes

Ingredients:

½ quart Heavy Cream

1 cup milk

1 Bay leaves

1 sprigs thyme

2 Tbsp, Boursin® Cheese

¼ cup crumbled Blue Cheese (optional)

2 cup white cheddar

3 Tbsp parmesan cheese

Lemon Juice, to taste

1 Pound Macaroni, cooked in salted water

16 oz rock shrimp, cleaned

6 oz Lump crab meat cleaned

Salt and Pepper to taste

Directions:

Combine heavy cream, milk, bay leaves, thyme and bring to boil

Let steep for 10 minutes

Strain

Add in cheeses one at a time allowing to melt before each addition (do not boil)

Adjust taste. Add in lemon juice and salt and pepper to taste

To Serve:

Sautee Shrimp in butter; add crab meat and fresh cooked pasta

Toss with desired amount of cheese sauce and finish with chopped parsley, salt and pepper to taste.

Recipe makes 8 Servings. All values are per serving. **Calories: 665**, Protein: 35g, Total Fat: 38g, Saturated Fat: 23g

THE PLAZA CAFE

Southampton, New York

Contributed by: Douglas Gulija

Restaurant Anecdotes

The Plaza Café is located in the heart of the Hamptons and has been serving New American Seafood for thirteen years. The restaurant is family run by Chef/proprietor Douglas Gulija and has been very fortunate to have received "Excellent" ratings by both The New York Times and Long Island Newsday. It has also been included in the Zagat Surveys America's Top Restaurants the past eight years.

We were very honored to be asked for a recipe for the Creative Calories & Recipes for Weight Gain Cookbook and decided that one of our desserts would be our best way to meet this request. We have provided a very simple but satisfying dessert that we hope you enjoy preparing at home for your family.

DESSERT CREATION

Created Especially for the Creative Calories Cookbook

Chocolate Bread Pudding with Caramelized Bananas and Peanut Butter Ice Cream

Includes:

Chocolate Brioche Pudding

Peanut brittle

Peanut butter ice cream

Carmalized bananas

Total Time: 2 ¼ hours plus freezing time for ice cream

Chocolate Brioche Pudding

Ingredients:

Brioche cubed 1 lb
Milk 3 cups
Heavy cream ¼ cup
Starbucks coffee liqueur ½ cup
Sugar 1 cup
Brown sugar 1 cup
Vanilla extract 1 Tbsp
Cocoa powder ¼ cup
Almond extract 2 tsp
Cinnamon 1 ½ tsp
Eggs, large beaten 6 ea
Chocolate, semisweet, chopped 8 oz

Directions:

Place bowl in ½ hotel pan
Whisk together milk, cream, liqueur
Combine both sugars with cocoa powder; add to milk mixture
Add extracts and cinnamon to eggs; combine with milk mixture
Add chocolate to milk mixture
Pour mixture over bread and let bread absorb for 20 minutes
Bake at 325° F for approximately 1 hour

Peanut Brittle

Ingredients:

Water 3 oz
Sugar 9 cups
Glucose 1 1/3 cups
Peanuts 3 cups

Directions:

Combine all but peanuts and heat to the caramel stage
Remove from heat and add peanuts
Pour onto silpat pad and cool
Process in robo coupe
Re-bake in desired shapes until reset

Peanut Butter Ice Cream

Yield: 1 quart

Ingredients:

Sugar ½ cup

Eggs 2 each

Peanut butter ½ cup

Cream 1 ½ cups

Milk 1 ½ cups

Directions:

Combine sugar and eggs

Add peanut butter

Add cream and milk

Process in machine

Presentation:

Cut out bread pudding with a ring mold, reheat and portion in center of plate

Slice a banana on the bias, dust with sugar and brulee with torch or under broiler

Arrange 3 pieces of bruleed banana around half the perimeter of the plate

Garnish the other half perimeter with dots of chocolate sauce and between each dot portion pieces of peanut brittle

Top bread pudding with peanut butter ice cream. Garnish plate with powdered sugar and fresh mint

The Plaza Café makes everything in-house at the restaurant including ice cream, peanut brittle, etc…

Recipe makes 8 servings. All values are per serving.

For Chocolate Bread Pudding: **Calories: 703,** Protein: 16 g, Total Fat: 23 g, Saturated Fat: 11 g

For Peanut Brittle (total recipe makes 16 servings of peanut brittle): **Calories: 656**, Protein: 14g, Total Fat: 13g, Saturated Fat: 2g

For Peanut Ice cream: **Calories: 343**, Protein: 8g, Total Fat: 28 g, Saturated Fat: 13 g

For Caramelized Banana: **Calories: 67,** protein: 0 g, Total Fat: 0 g, Saturated Fat :0 g

RISTORANTE
CAFÉ CORTINA

Farmington Hills, Michigan

Contributed By: Andrian Tonon

Restaurant Anecdotes

One of Michigan's best kept secrets is no longer a secret. Highly acclaimed by national and local media, this hidden gem continues to provide the simplicity of the purest Italian food. In the casual warm- toned setting, the seasoned staff guides guests through regional courses of 'antipasti, artisan pastas, risotto's, Mediterranean fish and Piedmont beef to ensure clients of a memorable experience. Only the highest quality ingredients, including produce from their on-premise garden enter the Tonon's kitchen back door. Summer or fall guests can dine on the beautiful ' Tuscan Patio' lush with grapevines and flowering trees or sit by the outdoor fireplace and enjoy a special dessert, a boutique grappa or expresso. Ristorante Café Cortina provides spaces for Business Meetings, Weddings, Anniversaries and all of life's special occasions.

Menu Selections

Zabaglione Mediterreano

Gnocchetti Di Casa Con Le Medaglioni Di Aragosta

Zabaglione Mediterreano

Total Time: 15 minutes

Ingredients

8 Egg yolks

1 cup Marsala

4 tsp sugar

4 tsp heavy cream

½ tsp finely chopped lavender

½ Tbsp of whipped mascarpone cheese

Directions:

Place all ingredients in stainless mixing bowl. Have a large pan of boiling water on the stove.

Place the stainless bowl in the larger pan and start whisking briskly, slowly add mascarpone until mixture becomes creamy golden should coat a spoon....
Serve in tall glasses and garnish with fresh lavender sprig

Recipe makes 4 Servings. All values are per serving **Calories: 229**, Protein: 2g, Total Fat: 14 g, Saturated Fat: 5 g

Cooking eggs till 160° F is suggested to ensure that they do not harbor salmonella.

Gnocchetti Di Casa Con Le Medaglioni Di Aragosta

Total Time: 90 minutes

Ingredients for Gnocchi:

Serves (4) (28 GNOCCHI)

5 Potatoes 4-6 lbs

½ cup flour

Salt to taste and water (can add nutmeg, basil)

Directions:

Peel, boil and drain (PBD Method)

Pass potatoes through Food Mill

Mix flour until dough ball consistency

Roll each out into desired thickness and length

Cut into small cubes, cut on slant to give bias appearance

Roll on Fork - - causes indentation to hold the sauce

Boil in salted water until they rise to the top of water

Drain Immediately

Ingredients for Sugo (Sauce):

Extra virgin olive oil 4 oz

Garlic ½ tablespoon

1 diced tomato

Saffron 2 tsp

Pepperoncini 1 tsp

Heavy Cream 3 cups

Directions for Sugo (Sauce):

Lightly sauté garlic in extra virgin olive oil

Add tomato, saffron, pepperoncini and last heavy whipping cream

Add gnocchi and sauté until desired consistency

Recipe makes 4 servings. All values are per serving. **Calories: 1296**, Protein: 16 g, Total Fat: 81 g, Saturated Fat: 43 g

six89

Carbondale, Colorado

Contributed By: Mark Fischer and Contributing Chef Bryce Orblom

Restaurant Anecdotes

Since 1998, Six89 has been considered one the most exciting and best restaurants in Colorado.

The award winning and trend setting "joint" continues to be a favorite for both locals and visitors, who enjoy the restaurants casual sophistication, simple décor and neighborhood feel.

Six89 features artisanal comfort food locally sourced whenever possible and seasonally based. The menu owes no particular allegiance to any cuisine but bears clear understanding of several. …lush by reason of ingredient, not frill.

Menu Selections

Lobster Corn Chowder

White Chocolate Chip Brownies

Lobster Corn Chowder

Total Time: 60 Minutes

Ingredients:

1 each red onion-diced fine

1 cup apple wood smoked bacon-julienne crosswise

1 Tbsp dry thyme

3 cup corn kernels-fresh

1 tsp crushed Red Pepper Flakes

2 quarts heavy cream

1 quart red potatoes – diced ¼"-blanched in salted water

2 each Jalapenos-seeded and diced fine

2 Tbsp lemon juice

Pinch cayenne

1 Tbsp Old Bay Seasoning®

2 Tbsp fresh thyme-chopped

1 Tbsp Kosher Salt

1 Tbsp fresh ground Black Pepper

4 cups fresh cooked Lobster Meat

Directions:

Sauté the bacon and the onion until the bacon is well rendered and crisp

While the bacon is rendering, blanch the potatoes until soft. Reserve

Add the thyme, corn, red pepper flakes, cream and return to a simmer

Add the blanched potatoes and stir. Return to a simmer

Add the peppers, lemon juice, house spice and fresh thyme. Adjust the seasonings

Add the lobster meat and heat through.

Serve. Garnish with fresh minced chives

Recipe makes 12 servings: All values are per serving. **Calories: 650,** Protein: 12 g, Total Fat: 59g, Saturated Fat: 37g

White Chocolate Chip Brownies

Total Time: 90 Minutes includes Baking time

Ingredients:

18 ounces butter-unsalted

12 ounces semi sweet chocolate chunks

12 ounces brown sugar

12 ounces granulated white sugar

1 teaspoon kosher salt

1 pint eggs – whole

1.5 oz cocoa powder-dutched

14 oz all purpose flour

14 oz white chocolate chunks

Directions:

Melt the butter and the semi sweet chocolate chunks, stirring until smooth in a double boiler

Allow to cool slightly

Prepare the pan by buttering and lining with parchment

Whisk together the sugars, salt and the eggs.

Sift together the flour and cocoa powder.

Add the flour mixture to the eggs and sugar and stir with a spatula just until combined.

Add the chocolate and stir further until just combined.

Fold in the white chocolate chips.

Place in 10 X 13 inch Baking dish and bake at 350° F approximately 60 minutes, turning after 15 minutes.

Cool

Recipe makes: 24 servings. All values are per serving. **Calories: 458**, Protein: 7g, Total Fat: 23g, Saturated Fat: 14g

Center Square, Pennsylvania

Contributed By: John Anderson, Executive Chef and Owner

Restaurant Anecdotes

John is one of the leading restaurateurs in the Philadelphia region, owning and operating several restaurants including Tequila Joe's in Oreland, Solaris Grille in Chestnut Hill and Center Square. How can he handle all of these successful restaurants? "Great staff, systems that work, and a love of what I'm doing." His passion, love and drive to provide the best dining experience for every guest is the key to his success.

House Penne

Total Time: 30 minutes

<u>**I**ngredients</u>:

Penne (6oz dry) cooked

Pancetta (small diced) 1 oz

Grilled chicken (sliced) 2.5 oz

16 to 20 Tiger shrimp (clean) 3 ea

Sautéed spinach ¼ cup

Red onion (sliced) 2 oz

Scallions 1 oz

White wine 2 oz

Heavy cream 4 oz

Asiago cheese (grated) 2 oz

<u>**D**irections</u>:

Preheat sauté pan, add pancetta and render fat

Add onions, shrimp and grilled chicken. Sauté for 1 minute

Add spinach allow it to wilt

Deglaze the pan with white wine and allow wine to burn off

Add pasta, cream, cheese and scallions allow to thicken (sauce should coat the pasta)

Season with salt and pepper

Recipe makes 4 servings. All values are per serving. **<u>Calories: 373</u>**, Protein: 16 g, Total Fat: 18 g, Saturated Fat: 11 g

Splendido

AT THE CHATEAU

Beaver Creek, Colorado

Contributed By: David Walford

Restaurant Anecdotes

Chef David Walford has been delighting diners at Splendido AT THE CHATEAU since 1994. His style of hearty but refined American cuisine is enhanced by his use of the freshest ingredients and cooking techniques such as wood fired ovens. He balances his respect for classic food traditions with an enthusiasm for unique foods and modern culinary challenges. His cuisine comes together in the warmth and tranquility of a French chateau overlooking Beaver Creek Village and the ski slopes.

Menu Selections

Mashed Potatoes

Splendido's Spicy Pecans

Potato Gnocchi, Toasted Garlic, Tomato, Basil and Guanciale

Lemon Blueberry Soufflé

Mashed Potatoes

Total Time: 40 minutes

Ingredients:

3 lb potatoes, russets

1 lb (4 sticks) butter, cold, diced up

1 cup whole milk

1 cup heavy cream

To taste sea salt

Directions:

Peel the potatoes and cut into 2 inch pieces.

Place in cold water with salt and bring to a boil.

Turn down heat and cook gently until just done, about 20 minutes or until a fork easily pierces them

Drain, immediately

Place in a single layer in a shallow pan and put in a 175° F oven to dry for about 5 minutes

Combine the milk and cream and bring to a simmer

Pass the warm potatoes through the fine holes of a food mill into a double boiler over simmering water

With a wooden spoon beat in the butter little by little

Then beat in the hot milk and cream

Season with salt

If the puree is too thick, add additional cream and/or milk

Recipe makes: 8 Servings. All values are per serving. **Calories: 687**, Protein: 6 g, Total Fat: 58 g, Saturated Fat: 37 g

Splendido's Spicy Pecans

Total Time: 15 minutes

Ingredients:

1 cup sugar

2 Tbsp Cayenne pepper

2 Tbsp dry mustard

2 Tbsp red pepper flakes

2 Tbsp powdered ginger

2 Tbsp cinnamon

8 cups pecan halves

Directions:

Mix all the spice ingredients together in a large mixing bowl

Blanch the pecans in boiling water for 30 seconds

Drain (don't allow to become dry) and then toss in the bowl with the spices until evenly coated

Deep fry at 350° F for about 1 minute until crispy, and then drain and cool on a sheet pan lined with paper towel

Serve as a snack or with cocktails

Recipe makes 18 servings. All values are per serving. **Calories: 373**, Protein: 4 g, Total Fat: 35 g, Saturated Fat: 3 g

Potato Gnocchi, Toasted Garlic, Tomato, Basil and Guanciale

Total Time: 2 hours

Ingredients for Gnocchi:

2 ½ pounds Russet potatoes (3 large potatoes)

2 Egg yolks

2 teaspoons Salt

1/8 tsp grated nutmeg

1½ cups flour (approximately)

Directions for Gnocchi:

Pre-heat the oven to 400° F and bake the potatoes in their skins for about 1 to 1 ½ hours or until they are completely cooked.

While the potatoes are still hot, cut them in half

Scoop out the flesh and pass through a food mill (ricer) into a large bowl

Add the egg yolks, salt and nutmeg to the potatoes and stir lightly.

Sprinkle in about ½ cup of the flour and work in gently with your hands.

The mixture will be quite sticky at this point

Add another ½ to ¾ cup of the flour and work in the flour gently so as not to knead the dough

Add a little more flour as necessary

The dough is done when it is slightly sticky, holds together when gently pressed together but is not at all dry

Form into a loaf shape and cover with a kitchen towel to prevent the dough from drying out while you are working with it.

Cut a fist sized chunk of dough off and with your hands gently roll into a rope about ½ to ¾ inches thick.

Cut the rope into pieces about ¾ inches, lightly dust with flour

Roll the pieces over a gnocchi paddle or over the back of a fork to create ridges if desired

With a spatula, gently transfer to a lightly floured sheet pan

Have ready a large pot of water boiling water with a strainer and prepare another pot filled with ice water

Cook the gnocchi, a few at a time in boiling water just until they have risen to the top.

Carefully remove with a slotted spoon or basket to an ice water bath and let cool briefly, then remove to a kitchen towel to drain

Place the gnocchi on an oiled sheet pan, cover and store in the refrigerator until needed (gnocchi may be frozen, in a single layer, then transferred to plastic bags and kept frozen)

Ingredients for Sauce:

4 oz Guanciale (pork Jowl), 1" pieces sliced thin (you can substitute pancetta)

¼ cup olive oil

¼ cup garlic cloves, sliced thin

¼ cup onion, diced fine

4 cups tomatoes, peeled, seeded and diced

1 Tbsp salt

1 tsp black pepper

¼ cup basil, sliced thin (chiffonade)

Directions for Sauce:

In a heavy bottomed 2 quart pot, cook the guanciale slowly in the olive oil over medium heat until lightly browned and crisp.

Drain, reserving the oil

Place the crisp guanciale on a plate lined with a paper towel and return the oil to the pot

Add the garlic to the reserved oil in the same pan and cook slowly over low heat, stirring constantly, watching very carefully until the garlic slices are nicely toasted.

Immediately add the onion to the browning garlic (otherwise the garlic will continue to cook and burn)

Cook over medium heat until the onion is beginning to lightly brown, stirring often

Add the tomatoes, season and simmer for about 6 to 8 minutes. Reserve warm.

To Serve:

Heat a 12 inch non-stick skillet over medium heat with 2 tablespoons of olive oil

In batches, lightly sauté the pre-cooked gnocchi until golden brown, being careful not to overcrowd the pan. This may take 2-3 batches.

Re-heat the sauce and add the basil and then ladle some of the warm sauce into each serving bowl.

Place the browned gnocchi on top of the sauce, grate fresh parmesan cheese over the gnocchi and then scatter the reserved crisp guanciale on top

Serve immediately

Recipe makes 6 main courses. All values are per serving. **Calories: 507**, Protein: 14 g, Total Fat: 17 g, Saturated Fat: 3 g

1 Tbsp Parmesan Cheese **Adds 22 calories**, 2g protein, 1g total fat, 1g saturated fat

Lemon-Blueberry Soufflé

Total Time: about 1 hour

Ingredients for Lemon- Blueberry Soufflé:

6-8 oz Soufflé dishes

11/3 cups egg whites, warm

½ cup Sugar

1 cup Lemon pastry cream, warm – see recipe below

6 Tbsp Fresh blueberries

12 tsp Grand Marnier liquor

12 tsp Confectioners' sugar

1½ Tbsp softened butter for preparing soufflé dishes

Directions for Lemon – Blueberry Soufflé:

Pre-heat the oven to 375° F

Prepare the soufflé dishes: Butter the insides and bottoms of the soufflé dishes with a thick layer of softened butter.

Dust the insides with granulated sugar and shake out the excess

Place the dishes on a sheet pan

Put the 1 cup of warm lemon pastry cream in a medium mixing bowl

Cover with plastic wrap and set aside

Place the warm egg whites into the bowl of an electric mixer

With the whip attachment, begin mixing on medium speed for 1 minute. Increase the speed to high and when the whites begin to get frothy, slowly add the sugar while continuing to whip

Whip until the whites are thick and glossy and holding soft peaks.

With a plastic spatula, fold the whites very gently into the bowl of the pastry cream (see recipe below)

Take the tray of soufflé dishes and place 1 Tbsp of blueberries in the bottom of each dish and 2 teaspoons of Grand Marnier on the blueberries.

Carefully spoon in the soufflé mixture to about ¼ to ½ inch from the top, leveling the tops off.

Gently tap the dishes on the countertop to settle the mix a little

Place the tray of soufflés on the center rack of a 375° F oven and bake for about 15 minutes until risen and firm

When finished the top should look slightly golden

Sprinkle with confectioner's sugar to finish and serve

Recipe makes 6 soufflés. All values are per soufflé. **Calories: 245**, Protein: 7g, Total Fat: 3g, Saturated Fat: 1g

Ingredients for lemon Pastry Cream:

1 ½ cup Whole Milk

1 lemon – just the yellow part of the peel removed with a peeler

¾ cup Granulated sugar

½ cup all purpose flour, sifted

3 Egg yolks

½ cup Fresh lemon juice, strained

¼ teaspoon salt

Directions for Lemon Pastry Cream:

In a medium stainless steel sauce pan, bring the milk and lemon peel to a simmer

Remove from heat and let stand for 10 minutes

Strain through fine strainer and return to the sauce pan and keep warm over low heat

Mix the sugar, sifted flour and salt together in a bowl and set aside

In a medium mixing bowl, beat the egg yolks with a whisk and gradually add the lemon juice and whisk until smooth

Gradually whisk the sugar/flour mixture into the egg mixture, whisking until smooth and continue beating until thick and lemony colored

Slowly whisk in half of the hot milk into the egg mixture in the mixing bowl, whisking thoroughly, then whisk in the remainder

Return this mixture back to the sauce pan and then over low heat bring to a simmer, whisking constantly with a wire whisk, until mixture is thick and holds a ribbon, about 5 minutes

Remove from the heat and scrape this mixture into the bowl of an electric mixer with a wire whip

Beat on high speed for four minutes

Set aside with plastic wrap on top to prevent a skin from forming

Recipe makes 2 cups. All values are per serving (for the amount of cream used for each soufflé). **Calories: 101g**, Protein: 2g, Total Fat: 2g, Saturated Fat: 1g

Cooking eggs till 160° F is suggested to ensure that they do not harbor salmonella. Soufflés can be served without lemon pastry cream or substituting whipped cream if desired.

Needham, Massachusetts

Contributed By: Dave Becker

Restaurant Anecdotes:

Sweet Basil is a fun B.Y.O. Italian Restaurant in Needham, Massachusetts. Of all the recipes that Sweet Basil prepares, this takes the cake as far as caloric intake. It is tasty, easy to make, and will stick to the ribs of all who eat this.

Rigatoni with Chicken, Broccoli, and Parmesan Cheese

Total Time: 50 Minutes

Ingredients:

1 stick of sweet unsalted butter

1 cup of white wine

1/3 cup of olive oil

1 lb of boneless, skinless chicken

1 bunch of broccoli

1 lb box of rigatoni cooked as per directions

5 cloves of garlic, minced

Grated parmesan cheese

Kosher Salt

Black Pepper

Directions:

Melt butter in deep skillet

Add oil and garlic

Simmer for about 15 minutes

Add wine and bring to a boil; then reduce heat to medium low for 20 minutes

Cut broccoli into small bite size pieces and steam in microwave for 8 minutes

Cut chicken into thin bite size pieces and cook in the butter, garlic and oil

Remove chicken when done and sauté broccoli in butter, garlic and oil for 5 minutes

Sprinkle broccoli with Parmesan cheese

Add cooked rigatoni to broccoli and chicken, and then season to taste with salt and pepper

Recipe makes 6 servings. All values are per serving. **Calories: 693**, Protein: 37g, Total Fat: 34g, Saturated Fat: 14g

Western Springs, Illinois

Contributed By: Paul Virant

Restaurant Anecdotes

The first restaurant in Western Springs to serve liquor since prohibition, Vie offers guests the opportunity to experience urban fine dining in a warm, relaxed village setting. Conveniently located steps from the Metra station, Vie attracts food-conscious diners from the entire Chicagoland area. Guests will find sanctuary in the intimate, gracious dining room housed in a two-story red brick building in the center of Norman Rockwell's Americana. Chef Virant's cuisine reflects the seasons, local harvests and the world becoming a smaller place. While the menu celebrates artisanal foods and local family farms, it also takes advantage of the increased availability of specialty foods from across the globe. Vie features Seasonal Contemporary American cuisine inspired by Western European cultures and rustic fare. Virant elevates familiar dishes by relying on the simplicity of a few, high-quality ingredients.

Almond Butter Cake

Total Time: 45 minutes

Ingredients:

500g (16.7 oz) Butter
500g (16.7 oz) Sugar
240g (8 oz) Yolks
250g (8.3 oz) All Purpose Flour
200g (6.7 oz) Almond Flour
200g (6.7 oz) Sliced Almonds

Directions:

Cream butter and sugar

Add yolks

Add dry ingredients and stir

Bake in a ½ sheet pan at 375°F for 20 minutes

Lower oven to 350°F and bake for another 20 minutes until a knife comes out clean

Recipe makes servings 36 squares. All values are per serving. **Calories: 220**, Protein: 2g, Total Fat: 15g, Saturated Fat: 7g

VIDALIA

An American Restaurant & Bar

1990 M ST. N.W. WASHINGTON, DC 20036

Contributed By: Chef R.J. Cooper

Slow Cooked Vidalia Onions

Total Time: 25 Minutes

Ingredients:

2 each Jumbo Vidalia onions

2 Tbsp Extra virgin olive oil

4 Tbsp unsalted butter

4 Tbsp Balsamic vinegar

1/3 cup Chicken stock or water

2 tsp fresh thyme, chopped

2 tsp fresh rosemary chopped

To taste salt and freshly ground pepper

½ cup Herbed-parmesan bread crumbs

1 cup Roasted chanterelle mushrooms

4 each aluminum foil squares "12x12"

Directions:

Peel the onions and cut in half horizontally.

Heat the oil and butter in a large covered skillet.

Add the onions and turn them once so that they are lightly browned and well coated with the cut side ending face up.

Season with salt and pepper; add the balsamic vinegar, stock or water, fresh herbs and cover.

Cook over very low heat, basting the onions with the liquid periodically until they are tender, about 15 to 20 minutes.

Remove the cover, turn the heat up to medium high and reduce the liquid in the pan until it coats the onion like a glaze. Adjust the seasoning, sprinkle with chopped fresh parsley and serve hot.

Recipe makes 4 Servings. All values are per serving. **Calories: 245**, Protein: 4g, Total Fat: 20g, Saturated Fat: 9g

THE WEST END GRILL

Ann Arbor, Michigan

Contributed by: Roland Pohlman

Restaurant Anecdotes

The West End Grill was opened in September of '95 and specializes in New American cuisine with Asian influences. With an emphasis on fresh seafood and steak items, the menu offers a variety of choices prepared in surprisingly unexpected ways. A small restaurant comprised of only 15 tables, the atmosphere is upscale, romantic, with servers reciting the menu from individual chalkboards placed at the table. Known as a "special occasion" restaurant, The West End Grill has been delighting customers, old and new, for almost 15 years.

Southwestern Crab Cakes

Total Time: 20 minutes

Ingredients:

¾ cup yellow onion chopped fine

½ cup celery chopped fine

2 Tbsp red pepper chopped fine

¾ cup mayonnaise

1 lb jumbo lump crab meat

1 Tbsp creole mustard (grocery store)

1 tsp cajun or blackening seasoning

1 dash of salt and white pepper

1 whole egg

½ cup Roasted corn (cut off kernel and place in oven to brown)

3 cups Panko Japanese bread crumbs

Butter for grilling

Directions:

Combine all ingredients (excluding Panko Bread Crumbs)

Mix thoroughly

Add Panko Bread Crumbs until mixture is firm but soft, not wet or dry

Form individual Crab Cakes

Place butter on a flat grill or hot pan

Sear Crab Cakes until brown on both sides

Recipe makes: 16 crab cakes. All values are per serving. **Calories: 244**, Protein: 12g, Total Fat: 23g, Saturated Fat: 6g

York
STREET

Dallas, Texas

Contributed By: Sharon Hage

Menu Selections

D*MN Good Brownies

Chocolate Soup

D*MN Good Brownies

Total Time: 30 minutes to prepare plus 30-35 minutes to bake

Ingredients:

1 cup sugar

¼ cup unsalted Butter

¼ cup water

½ lb (8 oz) bittersweet Chocolate Chips

1 teaspoon vanilla extract

2 eggs

1¼ cups All Purpose Flour

½ tsp Baking Powder

½ tsp salt

¼ cup Chocolate Chips

½ cup White Chocolate Chips

¾ cup Toasted Pecan Pieces

Directions:

Butter and Flour a "9x13" baking pan.

Set oven to 325° F

Boil butter, sugar and water in small sauce pan, stir in 8 ounces of bittersweet chocolate chips to melt.

Let this mixture cool.

Whip eggs and vanilla extract together in a separate bowl.

Sift together flour, baking powder, salt in separate bowl.

Fold egg mixture into cooled chocolate mixture.

Fold in flour mixture.

Fold in ¼ cup chocolate chips, white chocolate chips and ½ cup toasted pecans.

Spread into prepared pan.

Sprinkle with remaining ¼ cup toasted pecans.

Bake for approximately 30-35 minutes on middle shelf of pre-heated oven.

Toothpick inserted in center should come out with moist crumbs.

Let cool to room temperature and cut into 12 large squares.

Recipe makes 12 servings. All values are per serving. **Calories: 309**, Protein: 4g, Total Fat: 17g, Saturated Fat: 8g

Chocolate Soup

Total Time: 30 minutes

Ingredients:

1 ¼ cup whole milk

2 ¾ cup heavy cream

1/4 cup granulated sugar

1/8 tsp salt

½ tsp whole black peppercorns

2 pieces star anise

1 piece of cinnamon stick

1 tsp Earl Grey Tea

2 tsp vanilla extract

¼ cup coffee liqueur

6 oz high quality extra bittersweet chocolate, cut in small pieces

Directions:

In stainless steel sauce pan combine all ingredients except liqueur and chocolate

Bring mixture to a simmer, stirring occasionally

Remove mixture from the heat, cover tightly and let flavors infuse for one hour

In the meantime, melt chocolate pieces over a pot of barely simmering water, set aside uncovered, in a warm place

Bring milk mixture back up to a simmer, add the melted chocolate and whisk to combine thoroughly

Warm chocolate mixture on low heat 5 minutes

When mixture is completely incorporated, pour through a fine mesh strainer, discard solids

Whisk coffee liqueur into soup and serve warm topped with homemade marshmallows or biscotti

The soup may be prepared ahead up to 2 days and chilled. Re-heat over low heat before serving

Recipe makes 6 servings. All values are per serving. **Calories: 618**, Protein: 6g, Total Fat: 52g, Saturated Fat: 32g

Z

Cuisine

FRENCH BISTROT

Denver, Colorado

Contributed by: Patrick DUPAYS, Chef de Z Cuisine

Restaurant Anecdotes

Freshness, organic local produce, quality ingredients, and creativity are just a few words that come to mind when describing Z Cuisine.

Z Cuisine is a genuine French Parisian Bistrot and A' Côté is Denver's authentic French Absinthe Bar, located in the historic Highlands neighborhood - minutes from Lodo. We offer a daily 'blackboard"menu "cuisine du terroir" following the whispers of the seasons.

ColoRouge Tartiflette Fondue

Total Time: 35 minutes prep plus 25-35 to cook plus 30 minutes to preheat the oven

Ingredients:

2 lb organic fingerling potatoes or small potato

Sea salt

1 sprig rosemary or thyme

1/2 lb thick or regular cut bacon slices cut into ¼ inch piece

2 cloves fresh garlic, peeled and chopped super fine

2 cups of yellow onions, peeled and sliced thin

2 cups dry inexpensive white wine or white cooking wine

1 laurel leaf

2 whole MouCo ColoRouge cheeses (5.3 oz each) or any local cow milk cheese that will melt well. (feel free to ask for substitution if MouCo ColoRouge cheese is unavailable)

Ingredients for Crème Fraiche:

1 cup whipping cream

2 Tbsp buttermilk/non fat buttermilk

Directions for Crème Fraiche:

Mix whipping cream and buttermilk well.

Cover and let stand at room temperature for 24 hours or until thickened, then refrigerate.
(You could replace it by using 5 oz heavy whipping cream alone, or 1 cup of sour crème or pre-purchased crème fraiche at the store. This can be used directly from the refrigerator)

Directions for preparing:

Preheat oven to 375° F for 30 minutes

Wash and peel potatoes if necessary, leaving them whole

Place potatoes in boiling pot of salted water

Cook for 25 minutes or until tender

Pan fry the bacon in a non-stick skillet on a small/medium heat until crispy

When the bacon is fried and crispy, set it aside

Strain out excess bacon fat, keeping a tablespoon in the pan

Discard the rest of the bacon fat (do not discard in your sink, use an empty can for your left over fat and grease)

Using the same pan sauté the sliced onions on a medium heat for approximately 20 minutes or until golden brown, stirring and scraping the bottom of the pan

Then put the bacon back with the sautéed onions

Then deglaze the pan with 2 cups white wine, & 1 laurel leaf. Add the garlic and continue to cook for several minutes while stirring until all the ingredients are reduced and well combined becoming a sauce

Cut the boiled potatoes in thick slices 1/4 inch and mix them with the bacon, onions, white wine, garlic mixture

Portion the potato mixture into 4 individual ovenproof baking dishes

Slice the local cheese and spread it evenly on top of each individual baking dish

Spoon 1 Tbsp of crème fraiche over each dish

Bake for 25 - 35 minutes or until the cheese is melted and the top is lightly browned. don't overcook or the cheesy sauce will separate

Serve with a side salad

Voila, not too complicated

Best regards, **Patrick DUPAYS, Chef de Z Cuisine**:

Recipe makes 4 servings. All values are per serving. **Calories: 846**, Protein: 43, Total Fat: 48 g, Saturated Fat: 22g

Ann Arbor, Michigan

Contributed By: Ari Weinzweig

Zingerman's Delicatessen and Zingerman's Roadhouse

Provided by Ari Zingerman

Co-Founding partner of Zingerman's Community of Businesses

Recipes are excerpted from Zingerman's Guide to Better Bacon

Menu Selections

Bluefish-Fried in Bacon with Blue Grits

Hangtown Fry

Chocolate and Bacon Fat Gravy

Bluefish Fried in Bacon with Blue Grits

Recipe Anecdotes

Bluefish is one of my all-time favorite foods. But once you get off the East Coast it seems like hardly anyone knows it. This is a simple preparation, it has a great name, it's pretty eye-catching on the plate and, most importantly, it tastes extremely terrifically good. I made it with the really superb, organic, stone-ground blue grits that we get from Glenn Roberts' Anson Mills in South Carolina. Given that the old corn varieties ranged in color from white to red to yellow to blue and most everything in between (or even all on one cob—try Glenn's multi-colored "speckled grits" too!), blue grits really aren't all that strange. It'll mess up your all-blue color scheme, but this is also good with cooked greens on the side. To get back into the blue end of the spectrum you can follow with fresh blueberries and a dollop of fresh whipped cream (no bacon) for dessert! By Ari Weinzweig

Total Time: 1 Hour

Ingredients for the Grits:

Since the cooking time is the most challenging element of this recipe, I usually prepare a larger portion than I actually need and save some for later.

2 quarts cold water

1 pint Anson Mills blue grits (or some other high-quality brand)

1 tsp coarse sea salt

Directions for the Grits:

Heat the water in a heavy four-quart stockpot. Start mixing in the grits while the water warms up, stirring regularly—I find it infinitely easier to get lump-free grits this way. **A**dd salt and stir well.

Bring to a boil, then reduce the heat as low as possible. Stir a few more times, cover and cook on low for as long as you can—the long, slow cooking releases the starches and makes the grits really creamy. Once you get them cooking there's really nothing to do but stir every fifteen minutes or so.

Ingredients for the Fish:

When the grits are good and creamy and you're ready to eat, you can start the fish.

2 slices bacon, diced (I like the dry-cured Edwards' bacon for this one)

2 fillets fresh bluefish (2 lbs total)

Sea salt to taste

Freshly ground black pepper to taste

Olive oil (optional)

Directions for the Fish:

Fry the bacon in a heavy-bottomed skillet over moderate heat. Remove the bacon from the pan and drain, leaving the fat in the pan.

Pat the fish dry with a paper towel. Add the fish to the still-hot bacon fat in the skillet, skin side down (I think the skin is the best part!) Cook the fish until the skin is browned, then flip and cook quickly on the other side. If you need more fat, add a glug from your reserves or use a bit of olive oil.

While the fish is cooking, chop the bacon coarsely and set aside.

When the fish is almost done, put 1 cup cooked grits into 4 warm bowls. Place the fish on top, skin side down. Sprinkle the fat over the whole thing and top with salt, pepper and chopped bacon.

Recipe makes 4 Servings. All values are per serving. **Calories: 555**, Protein: 64 g, Total Fat: 17 g, Saturated Fat: 4g

Hangtown Fry
Recipe Anecdote

Oysters, eggs and bacon in one really good all-American dish, Hangtown Fry is a California classic. I love it because it is simple to make, it's delicious, and it's got a really great story to boot. I like to use a dry-cured bacon like Broadbent's because that's the sort of intense, long-cured bacon that Gold Rush-era cooks would likely have been working with.

The story of Hangtown Fry takes you to a northern California town originally known as Old Dry Diggins, then as Hangtown and now, Placerville. Back in Gold Rush days it was a prominent supply town – many of the area's miners went there to restock, cut loose and get themselves into a bit of trouble. The dish is said to have originated at the now-defunct El Dorado Hotel. Legend has it that a miner rolled into town with gold direct from a fresh strike and ordered the saloonkeeper to serve up his most special dish. The cook offered a choice of three high-end options: oysters, eggs (hard to transport and hence costly) or bacon. The miner told him to toss all three into one dish, and Hangtown Fry was born.

It's a versatile recipe – great for brunch, lunch or a light supper. Don't skimp on the egg quality – remember, they were a luxury in mid-nineteenth century Hangtown and remain a key component of the dish, not just a way to hold the oysters and bacon together.

Of course, you can vary the number of oysters according to how much gold you have in your pouch! By Ari Weinzweig

Total Time: 20 Minutes

Ingredients:

4 Tbsp oyster crackers, crushed

3 slices bacon, chopped

½ Tbsp bacon fat

3 oz fresh shucked oysters

3 large eggs, beaten

1/8 tsp sea salt

1/8 tsp freshly-ground Telicherry peppercorns

<u>Directions</u>:

Dredge the oysters in cracker crumbs. Leave them resting in the mix for at least 10 minutes so that the crumbs bond with the oysters.

In a non-stick skillet, cook the bacon over medium heat until crisp. Remove from the pan, leaving the bacon fat. Reduce the heat a bit and add the additional measure of fat.

When hot, add the oysters and cook for about 2 minutes, stirring gently, until the crumb coating is lightly browned.

Add the beaten eggs, salt and pepper, and stir gently. Cook over low heat, stirring softly ever thirty seconds or so, until the eggs are done as you like them.

Serve with San Francisco sourdough toast and "Folsom Prison Blues" playing in the background.

Recipe makes 1 generous or 2 smaller servings. All values are for 1 generous serving.

<u>Calories: 578</u>, Protein: 39g, Total Fat: 40 g, Saturated Fat: 11 g

Chocolate and Bacon Fat Gravy
Recipe Anecdotes

When I first read this recipe, I thought it was probably somewhere between a bad fad and a silly joke about Southern folk. But as silly or stupendous as the dish sounds, chocolate gravy is the real thing – a recipe with Appalachian roots, and a bit of strange and fascinating history. Most importantly, it actually tastes great.

How Appalachians started eating it, I can't say for sure; the dish's exact origins remain murky. Fred Sauceman, a professor of Appalachian Studies at East Tennessee State shared several theories. It could have some connection to traditional Mexican moles, which, of course, mix cacoa with savory and sweet into a sauce of this sort. Or perhaps it came up from the Spanish colonies on the East Coast. Fred's theory is that when an affordable Hershey's cocoa came to the hills in the twentieth century, people added it to gravy they were already making, adding sweetness and richness to lives that were not exactly replete with either (at least in a material, if not emotional sense). I can see chocolate gravy as a serious Sunday treat for poor kids in the hills.

The recipe below is a distillation of several that I got from Fred as well as John T. Edge and Angie Mosier of Southern Foodways Alliance. My bias towards darker chocolate and less sweetness got the recipe down to about half the milk it might have had in its original form. When it comes to the quality of cocoa, I use Scharffen Berger, which is darker than the more out-and-about Hershey's. You can, however, simply add more milk or use the Hershey's if you are after a mellower flavor.

Sara Roahan, who wrote the really good book Gumbo Tales, said "Those southerners really know how to eat. How much happier would my childhood have been with chocolate gravy? I cry to consider the answer." Make chocolate gravy, eat it and weep with joy. By Ari Weinzweig

Total Time: 30 Minutes

Ingredients:

4 slices dry-cured smoked bacon (I like the full-bodied intense flavor of Broadbent's or Benton's)

4 Tbsp bacon fat (rendered from the 4 slices plus any extra fat as necessary to bring it up to the full measure)

1 cup granulated white sugar

3 Tbsp all-purpose flour

¼ cup cocoa powder

1 cup whole milk

1 tsp sea salt

¼ tsp freshly-ground Tellicherry black pepper

Directions:

Fry the bacon in a heavy skillet over medium heat until crisp. Remove and drain on paper towels. Strain the fat and return 4 Tbsp worth back into the skillet. Keep the flame on low.

Combine the sugar, cocoa and flour in a bowl and mix well. Sift into the hot fat, stirring constantly until blended and the dry ingredients begin to melt into the bacon fat, about 3 to 4 minutes.

Chop the sliced bacon into small bits and set aside.

Slowly add a ¼ cup of the milk to the skillet, stirring constantly. The mixture will begin to bubble. Turn the heat up a touch and keep stirring until the sugar mixture is well dissolved. Slowly add the rest of the milk, a bit at a time, stirring throughout so that the gravy thickens—it should coat the spoon nicely. Add salt and pepper as above and the more to taste.

Spoon the hot gravy over warm buttered biscuits. (If you're in a pinch for time and find yourself biscuit-less, the gravy is good on white toast, too, although I don't think that's the mountain man way.) Crumble the bacon over the top and serve.

Recipe makes 8 Servings. All values are per serving. **Calories: 207**, Protein: 3g , Total Fat: 10g, Saturated Fat: 3g

Chapter 6 - Friendly Calories from Family and Friends

Tasty recipes from our wonderful friends and families are included in this chapter. These recipes include many child friendly dishes along with "tried and true weight gainers" used by individuals struggling to gain or maintain their body weight.

Appetizers

Cocktail Meatballs

Contributed By: Debbie Kaufman

Total Time: 30 Minutes

Ingredients:

2 lb chopped meat

1 egg

½ cup bread crumbs

½ tsp ginger

½ tsp garlic

1 tsp soy sauce

1 bottle (12 ounces) chili sauce

1 bottle (10 ounces) grape jelly

Juice of one lemon

¼ tsp olive oil

Directions:

Mix chopped meat with 1 egg, ½ cup bread crumbs, ¼ tsp ginger, ½ tsp garlic and 1 tsp soy sauce

Create small meatballs

Grease pan with olive oil

Bake meatballs 10 minutes, Turn and bake 5 minutes longer

Place chili sauce and grape jelly into pot. Cook and stir until jelly is melted

Place cooked meatballs into pot and cook 10 minutes longer

Serve meatballs with toothpicks and place sauce in bowl for dipping

Recipe makes 30 meatballs. All values are per serving. (3 meatballs). **Calories: 328**, Protein: 25g, Total Fat: 11g, Saturated Fat: 4g

Hot Spinach/Cheese Salsa Quiche

Contributed by: Robyn Goldberg

Total Time: 35 Minutes

Ingredients:

1 package frozen chopped spinach (defrosted)

1 bag shredded Mexican cheese

1 bar cream cheese (room temperature)

1 jar medium salsa

¼ cup heavy whipping cream

Directions:

Stir

Place in Baking Dish

Bake for 30 minutes at 350° F. Serve with chips (bake or microwave to reheat)

Recipe makes 6 servings. All values are per serving without chips. **Calories: 349**, Protein: 15 g, Total Fat: 30 g, Saturated Fat: 19 g

Pesto and Sun Dried Tomato Torte

Contributed By: Wendi Tepper

Total Time: 20 Minutes plus overnight refrigeration

Ingredients:

2 cups pesto

4 oz soft goat cheese

8 oz cream cheese

¼ cup pine nuts

¼ cup thin sliced sun-dried tomatoes (oil packed and drained)

8 or 9 slices provolone cheese

Directions:

Line a loaf pan with plastic wrap, both horizontally and vertically

Mix goat and cream cheese until smooth

Layer as follows: 3 slices provolone cheese in the bottom of the loaf pan, then ½ goat/cream cheese, pesto sauce, pine nuts, sundried tomatoes

Layer 2-3 slices of provolone

Spread remaining goat/cream cheese, pesto sauce, pine nuts, sundried tomatoes

Top with last 3 slices of provolone cheese

Cover and refrigerate overnight

Unfold mixture, invert and place on plate

Serve with sliced French bread or crackers

Notes;

This can be frozen

Recipe makes 12 servings. All values are per serving (without bread or crackers).
Calories: 378, Protein: 13g, Total Fat: 32g, Saturated Fat: 14g

Beef Nachos Supreme

Contributed By: Nadine Cohen

Total Time: 60 minutes

Ingredients for Salsa:

16 oz Prepared Salsa

Ingredients for Refried Beans

½ cup canned re-fried beans

1 oz pepper Jack cheese, shredded (about ¼ cup)

1 Tbsp chopped canned pickled jalapeno chilies

Ingredients for Beef

2 Tbsp Canola oil

1 small onion, minced

3 garlic cloves, minced

1 Tbsp chili powder

1 tsp ground cumin

½ tsp dried oregano

1 tsp salt

1 lb 93% lean ground beef

2 Tbsp Tomato Paste

1 Tbsp Brown Sugar

10 oz can Chipotle Chile in Adobo Sauce, chopped, sauce reserved

½ cup water

2 Tbsp fresh lime juice

Ingredients for Assembly

6 oz yellow tortilla chips,

3 oz blue tortilla chips

1 lb pepper jack cheese, shredded (4 cups)

3 jalapeno chilies, sliced into thin rings

Optional ingredients: Sour Crème, 1 diced avocado, Cilantro leaves

Directions for the beans

Pulse all the ingredients in the food processor until smooth. Transfer to a bowl and cover with plastic.

Directions for the beef

Heat the oil in a large skillet over medium heat until simmering.

Cook the onion, stirring occasionally, until softened, about 4 minutes.

Add the garlic, chili powder, cumin, oregano, and salt and cook until fragrant, about one minute.

Add the beef and cook, breaking the meat into small bits with a wooden spoon and scraping the pan bottom to prevent scorching, until no longer pink, about five minutes.

Add the tomato paste, sugar, chili, and adobo sauce and cook until the paste begins to darken, about one minute.

Add the water, bring tomatoes to a simmer and cook over medium-low until the mixture is nearly dry, 5-7 minutes.

Stir in the lime juice and transfer the mixture to a plate lined with several layers of paper towels. Use more paper towels to blot up excess grease and discard.

To assemble adjust an oven rack to the middle position and heat the oven to 400° F

Spread half of the chips on a large, oven safe serving platter or a 13x9inch baking dish.

Dollop half of the bean mixture over the chips, then spread evenly. Scatter half of the beef mixture over the beans, top with 2 cups of the cheese and half of the jalapeños.

Repeat with the remaining chips, beans, beef, cheese and jalapeños. Bake until the cheese is melted and just beginning to brown, 12 to 14 minutes. Top with the salsa and garnish with sour cream, avocado and cilantro leaves if desired.

The salsa, re-fried beans, and beef can be refrigerated in separate containers for up to one day and assembled as above before eating.

Recipe makes 8 servings. All values are per serving. **Calories: 568**, Protein: 32g, Total Fat: 36g, Saturated Fat: 16g

Main Dishes

Baked Macaroni and Cheese

Contributed By: Ruth Blumenfeld

Total Time: 35 Minutes

Ingredients:

3 cups dry macaroni

¾ cup milk

1½ tsp salt

12 oz sour cream

2 cups grated cheddar cheese

1 egg (beaten)

1 stick butter/margarine (softened)

Directions:

Preheat oven to 375° F

Cook macaroni according to directions on package and drain

Mix butter, milk, sour cream, and cheese in large bowl

Add cooked/drained macaroni

Add beaten egg to mixture

Pour into baking dish

Bake 20 minutes (leftovers taste good the next day, too)

Recipe makes 6 servings. All values are per serving. **Calories: 649**, Protein: 20g
Total Fat: 43g, Saturated Fat: 24g

Blintz Souffle

Contributed By: Barbara Reiff

Total Time: 1 Hour and 15 Minutes

Ingredients for Batter:

½ cup sugar

2 eggs

1 cup Flour

¼ tsp Baking Powder

¼ cup whole milk

1 tsp vanilla

1 stick of butter, melted

Ingredients for Filling:

2 Pounds Whole Milk Ricotta Cheese

2 Eggs

¼ cup Sugar

1 Tbsp Lemon Juice

Directions:

Mix batter in medium bowl

Mix filling in large bowl

Grease 9 X 13" Casserole

Pour ½ of batter into casserole

Spread filling over batter

Cover with remaining batter

Bake for 1 hour @ 300° F

Recipe makes 6 servings. All values are per serving. **Calories: 629**, Protein: 24g, Total Fat: 39g, Saturated Fat: 24g

Bourek

Contributed By: Barbara Reiff

Total Time: 40 Minutes

Ingredients:

1 Stick of butter, melted

½ cup milk

1 package frozen chopped spinach, thawed and drained

8 ounces shredded mozzarella cheese

1 Package phyllo dough

1 Egg

Non-fat Dried Milk (optional)

Directions:

Mix milk and butter

Layer phyllo sheets in greased 9 X 12″ baking dish and brush every other sheet with the milk/butter mixture.

When ½ the sheets are used, spread ½ the cheese over the pan

Put one more sheet over cheese

Spread spinach

One more sheet

Spread remaining cheese

Continue to layer the sheets and brush with milk/butter mixture

When all of the sheets are layered, beat egg into remaining milk/butter mixture and pour over the top of the casserole.

Bake at 375° F for 25 minutes

Recipe makes 6 servings. All values are per serving. **Calories: 530**, Protein: 17g, Total Fat: 28g , Saturated Fat: 16g

Chicken Alfredo

Contributed By: Michael Franklin

Total Time: 50 Minutes

Ingredients:

2 boneless, skinless chicken breasts
2 eggs
¼ cup milk
½ cup grated parmesan cheese
1 Tbsp parsley
⅓ cup bread crumbs
4 slices mozzarella cheese

Ingredients for sauce:

3 tbsp butter
½ pint heavy cream
½ cup milk
½ cup grated parmesan cheese
1 Tbsp parsley

Directions:

Beat eggs with milk
Mix in ½ cup grated parmesan cheese and parsley
Dip chicken pieces in egg mixture and roll in bread crumbs
Lightly brown chicken in a skillet with a bit of olive oil and remove to baking dish

Directions for sauce:

Preheat oven to 350° F and over medium heat, melt butter
Add cream and milk, stirring constantly
Add cheese and parsley until it is a warm sauce
Pour sauce over chicken breasts
Cover with foil and bake for 20 to 30 minutes or until chicken is cooked
During the last five minutes, add a slice of mozzarella to each piece of chicken and allow it to melt

Recipe makes 2 servings. All values are per serving. **Calories: 1027**, Protein: 58g, Total Fat: 81g, Saturated Fat: 47g

Chicken, Zucchini and Avocado Tortillas

Contributed By: Debbie Kaufman

Total Time: 10 Minutes

Ingredients:

2 Zucchinis (sliced thin long strips)

2 Multi Grain Flour Tortillas

1 egg white

½ cup Panko Crumbs

1 Cup Chicken (white meat roasted chicken (could be store bought: cut into thick strips)

½ Avocado

½ cup Shredded cheese

Optional: For Dipping: Salsa, Sour Cream

Directions:

Coat zucchini with egg white

Place panko crumbs on top of zucchini

Place strips of zucchini in a rimmed dish with ½ cup water on the bottom

Microwave for about 10-15 minutes until zucchini cooks and softens

Warm chicken in the microwave

Warm tortilla 45 seconds in a pan and flip

Once flipped, place ½ cup of shredded cheese down the center of each tortilla and continue to heat for 45 seconds

Place warm tortillas with melted cheese on a plate and place warm chicken and zucchini down the center of each

Placed sliced avocado on top of the chicken, zucchini and cheese on each tortilla

Roll each and slice in half

Serve with 2 T Sour cream and 2 T Salsa for dipping

Recipe makes 2 Tortillas. All values are per serving. **Calories: 869**, Protein: 36g, Total Fat: 44g, Saturated Fat: 18g

French Salisbury Steak with Garlic Cheese Toasts

Contributed By: Debbie Kaufman

Total Time: 45 Minutes

Ingredients:

1 ¼ lb ground chuck

¼ cup fresh minced parsley

2 Tbsp scallion minced

1 tsp kosher salt

½ tsp black pepper

2 Tbsp flour

1 Tbsp olive oil

2 cup onions, sliced

1 tsp sugar

1 Tbsp garlic, minced

1 Tbsp tomato paste

2 cup beef broth

¾ tsp kosher salt

½ tsp dried thyme leaves

Directions:

Combine ground chuck, parsley, scallion, salt and pepper

Divide evenly into 4 portions and shape each into ¾" patties

Place 2 Tbsp flour in a shallow dish; dredge each patty in flour; reserve 1 tsp flour

Heat 1 Tbsp oil in a sauté pan over medium-high heat

Add patties and sauté 3 minutes on each side, or until browned. Remove from pan

Add onions and sugar to pan

Sauté 5 minutes

Stir in garlic and tomato paste; sauté 1 minute or until paste begins to brown

Sprinkle onions with reserved flour; cook 1 minute

Stir in broth and add the salt and thyme

Return meat to pan and bring soup to a boil

Reduce heat to medium-low, cover and simmer 10 minutes

Serve over Garlic cheese toasts (see next page)

Recipe makes 4 Servings. All values are per serving. **Calories: 450**, Protein: 36g, Total Fat: 27g, Saturated Fat: 10g

Garlic Cheese Toasts

Contributed By: Debbie Kaufman

Total Time: 5 Minutes

Ingredients:

4 slices whole wheat bread

4 tablespoons parmesan cheese

4 tsp garlic powder

2 tablespoons butter

Directions

Place butter on bread

Sprinkle bread with garlic and parmesan cheese

Bake or toast

Recipe makes 4 toasts. All values are per toast. **Calories: 149** Protein: 5g, Total Fat: 9g, Saturated Fat: 5g

French Toast Casserole

Contributed By: Michelle Shaer

Total Time: 80 Minutes

Ingredients for French Toast Casserole

1½ Cup Brown Sugar

1 stick unsalted butter, melted

1½ tsp cinnamon

2 small loaves Pepperidge Farm® white bread, remove crust

6 large eggs

2 cup whole milk

1 Tbsp vanilla extract

2 sliced bananas

Maple Syrup

Directions:

Combine melted butter and brown sugar and cinnamon and spread evenly on bottom of 9 X 12 inch baking dish

Arrange white bread slices in 2 layers over mixture, packing them in tightly

Whisk eggs, milk, vanilla extract together

Optional - arrange banana slices over bread

Pour egg mixture over bread

Cover baking dish with aluminum foil

Refrigerate overnight

Bring to room temperature, approximately 20 minutes before baking

Bake at 350° F for about 45 minutes, and until lightly browned

Remove from oven and top with 2 Tbsp maple syrup

Recipe makes 6 servings. All values are per serving. **Calories: 866**, Protein: 19g, Total Fat: 28g, Saturated Fat: 14g

Individual Pizzas for kids to help make

Contributed By: Carol Day

Prep Time: 20 Minutes

Directions:

Toast an English muffin

Put tomato sauce on the English muffin

Put grated mozzarella cheese on top of the sauce

Top with your favorite topping … pieces of chicken, pepperoni, sausage

Bake in the oven @ 350° F until sauce is hot and cheese is melted

Recipe makes 1 serving. All values are per serving. **Calories: 312,** Protein: 17g, Total Fat: 14g, Saturated Fat: 8g

Additional toppings

1 ounce grilled chicken adds 47 calories, 9g protein, 1g fat, 0g saturated fat

1 ounce pepperoni adds 132 calories, 6g protein, 11g total fat and 5g saturated fat

1 ounce sausage adds 96 calories, 6g protein, 8g total fat, 3g saturated fat

Linguine with Tomatoes and Basil

Contributed By: Linda Weber

Total Time: 20 minutes / Prepare mixture 2 hours before serving

Ingredients:

4 Large ripe tomatoes, cut in ¼-in cubes

1 lb Brie cheese, rind removed, torn in irregular pieces

1 cup cleaned fresh basil, cut into strips

3 cloves garlic, minced

1 cup plus 1 Tbsp olive oil

2 ½ tsp salt

½ tsp fresh ground pepper

1½ lb linguine

Directions:

Combine tomatoes, Brie, basil, garlic, 1 cup olive oil, ½ teaspoon salt and pepper in large bowl

Prepare at least 2 hours before serving and set aside at room temperature

Boil 5 quarts water

Add 1 Tbsp olive oil and remaining salt

Boil linguine until tender, 8-10 minutes

Drain pasta and toss immediately with sauce

Serve with fresh pepper and grated parmesan cheese

Recipe makes 8 servings. All values are per serving. **Calories: 698** Protein: 23 g, Total Fat: 47 g, Saturated Fat: 15 g

Mac & Cheese Recipe

Contributed By: Vanessa Feinsod

Total Time: 55 Minutes

<u>Ingredients:</u>

1 Tbsp butter

2 Tbsp flour

2 cup shredded cheddar cheese

2 cup milk

Box of elbow macaroni or medium shells

Wheat germ or bread crumbs to top

<u>Directions</u>:

In a medium sauce pan, melt the butter

As the butter is melting, whisk in the flour, and as it thickens, add the milk

Let stand for about 5 minutes until the milk starts to get thicker, occasionally stirring

After the milk thickens, slowly add in the cheese.

While you are making the cheese sauce, make pasta according to the box

Once pasta and sauce are finished cooking, combine in a bowl.

Put in the oven at 350° F for 30-45 minutes. Before baking, sprinkle either bread crumbs or wheat germ on the top.

<u>Recipe makes</u> 6 servings. All values are per serving. **<u>Calories: 526</u>**, Protein: 23g, Total Fat: 19g, Saturated Fat: 11g

Noodle/Spinach Casserole

Contributed By: Jan Zauzmer

Prep Time: 45 Minutes

Ingredients:

8 Tbsp flour

8 Tbsp butter

3 cup whole milk

Several dashes of salt

2 boxes frozen spinach

1 lb. broad egg noodles

2 jars drained pimientos

Directions:

Melt flour and butter over very low heat on burner

Add milk and salt and cook over low heat stirring with whisk until sauce thickens

Add flour if thin

Cook and drain spinach

Boil and drain noodles

Then combine spinach, noodles, pimientos, and cream sauce for a rich side dish

Recipe makes 10 servings. All values are per serving. **Calories: 345**, Protein: 11g, Total Fat: 15g, Saturated Fat: 8g

Pasta with Sausage in Tomato Cream Sauce

Contributed By: Stacy Kamisar

Total Time: 25 Minutes

Ingredients:

1 lb spicy sausage, casing removed

1 35 oz can of plum tomatoes, quickly pureed

1 cup chicken broth

1-2 Tbsp tomato paste

½ cup heavy cream

1 cup frozen peas

1 pound penne

½ Cup parmesan cheese

Directions:

Sauté sausage in pan until brown, crumbling with fork

Add tomatoes, paste and chicken broth and simmer ten minutes while pasta is cooking

Add cream stirring until combined

Add frozen peas and cook until tender

Drain pasta and add to sauce

Season with parmesan cheese and serve

Recipe makes 4 servings. All values are per serving **Calories: 604**, Protein: 43g, Total Fat: 23g , Saturated Fat: 12g

Sharon's Dairy Kugel

Contributed By: Sharon Shylit

Total Time: 1 Hour and 10 Minutes

Ingredients:

1 Bag wide noodles, cooked and drained

1 tsp Cinnamon

16 oz Sour Cream

16 oz Cottage cheese, small curd

8 oz cream cheese

4 Eggs

1 Cup Sugar

Directions:

Blend the last 5 ingredients with electric mixer until smooth and creamy

Mix in Noodles

Pour into 9 X 13 Baking Dish

Sprinkle Cinnamon over top

Bake @ 350° F for 1 hour

Recipe makes 6 servings. All values are per serving. **Calories: 837**, Protein: 29g, Total Fat: 39g, Saturated Fat: 22 g

Shepherd's Pie

Contributed by: Debbie Kaufman

Total Time: 55 Minutes

Ingredients

1 ½ lbs lean ground beef

1 package brown gravy

1 cup of water

1 tsp Worcestershire sauce

2 cups mashed potatoes

1 Tbsp butter or margarine

½ cup sour cream

¼ cup shredded Cheddar cheese

¼ cup shredded Mozzarella cheese

Directions:

Heat oven to 350° F

Cook the ground beef in a skillet over medium heat until meat is browned, about 5-10 minutes

Add the packet of gravy, water, Worcestershire sauce and simmer on low to medium heat for 2 minutes

Separately, combine mashed potatoes with butter or margarine and sour cream

Pour meat mixture into a 9 inch pan. Spread mashed potatoes over the meat mixture and top with grated cheeses.

Bake for 15-20 minutes, until heated through

Recipe makes 4 servings. All values are per serving. **Calories: 696**, Protein: 43g, Total Fat: 35g, Saturated Fat: 16g

String Pie

Contributed By: Carol Day

Total Time: 45 Minutes

Ingredients:

1 pound ground beef or chicken

½ cup chopped onion if desired

¼ cup chopped green pepper if desired

1 jar (15 1/2 ounces) spaghetti sauce

8 oz spaghetti, hot cooked and drained

½ cup grated Parmesan cheese

2 eggs, beaten

2 tsp butter

1 cup cottage cheese or ricotta cheese

1 cup shredded mozzarella cheese

Directions:

Cook meat, onion and green pepper in large skillet over medium-high heat until meat is brown, stirring to separate meat into small pieces. Drain fat

Stir in spaghetti sauce, mix well

Combine spaghetti, Parmesan cheese, eggs and butter in a large bowl, mix well. Place in the bottom of a 13 x 9" pan

Spread cottage or ricotta cheese over top

Pour sauce mixture over cheese

Sprinkle mozzarella cheese over top

Bake in preheated 350° F oven until cheese melts, about 20 minutes

Recipe makes 6 servings. All values are per serving. **Calories: 462**, Protein: 31g, Total Fat: 27g, Saturated Fat: 12g

The Ultimate Grilled Cheese Sandwich

Contributed By: Evelyn Scher

Total Time: 15 Minutes

Ingredients:

4 slices white bread

2 slices mozzarella cheese

2 slices cheddar cheese

2 slices American cheese

1 stick unsalted butter (1/4 lb)

Pinch of salt

Directions to assemble sandwiches:

Lay out two slices of white bread

Place one slice of each cheese on each of the two bread slices in the following order: American, cheddar and mozzarella

Top off with the remaining slices of white bread.

In a large frying pan over medium high heat, melt the unsalted butter. Add a pinch of salt and place the assembled sandwiches in the pan

Allow the sandwiches to pan fry for about 3 minutes on each side or until cheeses have fully melted and bread turns golden brown

Make sure to use a spatula to press down and flatten the sandwiches.

This will make the cheeses ooze slightly to create the ultimate cheese sandwich

Makes 2 sandwiches

Recipe makes 2 servings. All values are per serving. **Calories: 855**, Protein: 23g, Total Fat: 73g, Saturated Fat: 45g

Side Dishes

Broccoli Casserole

Contributed By: Michael Franklin

Total Time: 45 Minutes

<u>Ingredients</u>:

2 lbs broccoli crowns (fresh or frozen)

8 slices of bacon – cooked

10 oz of Sour Cream

8 oz of mild cheddar cheese - grated

<u>Directions:</u>

Preheat oven to 350° F

Cook the broccoli

Lay the hot, cooked broccoli into an 8 X 10-inch baking dish.

Evenly place the cooked bacon on top of the broccoli

Spread the sour cream over the bacon

Sprinkle the cheese on top of the sour cream

Bake for 20-30 minutes or until the cheese is melted

Recipe makes 4 servings. All values are per serving. **<u>Calories: 549</u>**, Protein: 28g, Total Fat: 42g, Saturated Fat: 24g

Cream of Spinach

Contributed By: Evelyn Scher

Total Time: 20 Minutes

Ingredients:

1 Tbsp olive oil

2 cloves garlic, crushed

2 lb frozen chopped spinach

2 cup heavy cream

1 cup parmesan cheese, grated

Salt and pepper to taste

Directions:

In a deep frying pan, heat olive oil over medium high heat

Add the crushed garlic and spinach

Using a wooden spoon, stir the spinach to incorporate garlic and olive oil; then cover pan

Let spinach cook for about 8-10 minutes or until fully wilted and reduced.

Uncover pan and add the heavy cream and parmesan cheese

Stir with wooden spoon and let the cream come to a boil

Reduce heat to medium-low, cover the pan

Once again, let the cream of spinach mixture simmer for another 3 minutes

Season to taste and serve with more grated parmesan cheese

Recipe makes 6 servings. All values are per serving. **Calories: 402**, Protein: 13g, Total Fat: 36g, Saturated Fat: 21g

Cream Soups

Contributed By: Evelyn Scher

Total Time: 30 Minutes

Ingredients:

2 Tbsp flour

2 Tbsp butter

1 cup of cooked diced or mashed vegetable

1½ cup milk

Pinch of salt

Variations:

ASPARAGUS – Cut tender stalks and tips (1/2 inch thick)

BROCCOLI – cut or chop fine, using some leaf sections

CELERY – cut fine, including small bit of leaves

CORN – cut from cob or use cream style canned corn

MUSHROOMS – cut tender part of stems with tops (very fine)

MUSHROOM AND POTATO – add equal amount of potato, diced fine

POTATO – dice – stir while cooking

SPINACH – chop carefully – well washed leaves

TOMATO – peel fresh whole tomatoes or used canned varieties – dice well

Directions:

Blend melted butter and flour in a saucepan over moderate heat, rubbing with back of spoon till smooth but not brown

Stir in milk slowly and cook one minute

Add salt and 1 cup of cooked, diced or mashed vegetable

Bring to a slow boil

Stir while cooking to prevent skin from forming

SUGGESTED FLAVORINGS FOR SOUPS:

1 Tbsp minced onion browned in 1 tablespoon butter

Grated American cheese sprinkled on top before serving

1 tsp lemon juice plus 1 tablespoon brown sugar for tomato soup

Browned croutons

Chopped hard cooked egg yolks

Recipe makes 2 servings. All values are per serving. (Nutrient calculations are based on soup made with 1 cup of cooked broccoli. Other vegetables yield similar nutrient values). **Calories: 272**, Protein: 9g, Total Fat: 19g, Saturated Fat: 11g

Exotic Salad

Contributed By: Alison Kallenbach

Total Time: 15 Minutes

Ingredients:

1 hearts of romaine lettuce

½ cup slivered almonds

2 Tbsp chopped yellow pepper

½ cup crumbled feta cheese

½ cup sliced avocado pieces

½ cup sea salt and pepper croutons

½ cup Craisins®

7 Tbsp Marzetti Simply Dressed® Balsamic all natural vinaigrette

Directions:

Grease aluminum foil and toast ½ cup slivered almonds for 4 minutes at 350° F

Cut up hearts of romaine lettuce into small pieces

Place the following ingredients into salad bowl and toss: romaine lettuce, toasted slivered almonds, yellow pepper, feta cheese and craisins

Add the avocado, croutons and balsamic vinaigrette dressing right before serving.

Recipe makes 4 servings. All values are per serving. **Calories: 505**, Protein: 9g, Total Fat: 35g, Saturated Fat: 5g

Layered Lettuce

Contributed By: Antoinette Calabro

Total Time: 20 Minutes

Ingredients:

1 head of iceberg lettuce

4 to 5 scallions

Celery

1 green pepper

10 oz package of frozen peas (defrosted and drained)

1 cup Hellman's® mayonnaise

½ cup sour cream

½ packet ranch style dressing

½ cup shredded cheddar cheese

4 strips cooked bacon (crumpled)

21/2 tsp sugar

Directions for Salad:

Layer the following and sprinkle with 2 to 3 tsp of sugar

1 head of iceberg lettuce (torn)

4 or 5 scallions (cut in pieces)

½ cup finely chopped celery

½ cup finely chopped green pepper

1 (10 ounce) package of frozen peas

In a separate bowl, mix the following ingredients:

1 cup Hellman's® mayonnaise

½ cup sour cream

½ packet ranch style dressing

Layer this mixture of top of the salad and sprinkle cheddar cheese and crumbled bacon.

Recipe makes 4 servings. All values are per serving. **Calories: 629**, Protein: 12g, Total Fat: 56g, Saturated Fat: 14g

Mozzarella Sticks

Contributed By: Evelyn Scher

Total Time: 30 Minutes to prepare, plus time for freezing

Ingredients:

1 ½ cups bread crumbs

16 ounces block mozzarella cheese cut into ½ - ¾" thick pieces

4 large eggs, beaten

3 cups flour

1 ½ cups vegetable oil

Directions:

Place flour, eggs and bread crumbs in separate bowls and put them on the counter in that order

Dip the cheese stick in the flour and coat completely

Dip the cheese stick into the eggs, submerging them completely

Dip the cheese stick into the breadcrumbs

Use your hands to coat completely

Dip the breaded cheese stick once again into the eggs, and once more into the bread crumbs

You should have a thickly coated cheese stick

Repeat process with remaining sticks

Cover and freeze until frozen, about 2 hours or up to 2 days

Heat oil in large frying pan over medium heat

Fry the breaded cheese sticks in batches, until golden brown, about 2 minutes

Serve with dipping sauce, e.g. marinara sauce

Note: When frying, watch for cheese bubbling out of the breadcrumbs coating.... If any escapes, remove immediately from oil

Recipe makes 22 Mozzarella sticks. All values are per serving. (2 Mozzarella sticks)

Calories: 424, Protein: 15g, Total Fat: 27g, Saturated Fat: 7g

Orzo and Scallion Pilaf

Contributed By: Alison Rosenberg

Total Time: 30 Minutes

<u>Ingredients</u>:

½ stick butter

2 bunches scallions finely chopped

1 cup orzo

3 cups jasmine rice

1 49 ounce can chicken broth

Salt/pepper to taste

<u>Directions</u>:

Melt butter in heavy saucepan over medium heat

Add scallions and sauté for about 3-5 minutes

Add orzo and brown slightly

Add rice and broth

Season to taste

Bring everything to a boil and reduce heat to low

Cover and cook for 20 minutes

Remove from heat and wait 5 minutes

Fluff with a fork and serve

Recipe makes 8 servings. All values are per serving. **<u>Calories: 207</u>**, Protein: 4g, Total Fat: 8g, Saturated Fat: 3g

Pumpkin Soup

Contributed By: Stacy Kamisar

Total Time: 45 Minutes

Ingredients:

2 Tbsp unsalted butter

2 stalks celery, diced

1 carrot, diced

1 onion, diced

2 Tbsp flour

1 15 oz can pumpkin puree

4 cups chicken broth

1 cup heavy cream

Nutmeg

Salt

Pepper

Directions:

Sauté onion in butter until translucent and add celery and carrot until lightly browned

Remove from heat and add flour

Return to heat and add pumpkin and chicken broth

Simmer 30 minutes

Puree with hand-held blender

Add cream and heat until incorporated

Season with nutmeg, salt and pepper

Recipe makes 6 servings. All values are per serving. **Calories: 238**, Protein: 3g, Total Fat: 21g , Saturated Fat: 12g

Potato Pancakes

Contributed By: Debbie Kaufman

Total Time: 45 Minutes

Ingredients:

6 potatoes

1medium onion

1 teaspoon salt

1 egg beaten

3 tablespoons flour

½ teaspoon baking powder

Vegetable Oil

Apple sauce or Sour cream

Directions:

Finely grate potatoes and 1 medium onion

Combine potatoes and onion mixture with salt, egg, flour and baking powder

Cover bottom of pan with 1/8" of oil and heat on medium high or until a small amount of mixture sizzles when placed in heated oil

Place 1 Tbsp of the potato mixture into the pan, one at a time until the pan is filled with space in between each pancake.

Fry about 4 minutes. Turn and flatten pancakes. Continue to fry another 3-4 minutes until golden brown on each side

Take out the pancakes and place batch on a paper towel

Continue to fry the rest of the pancake mixture and repeat

Serve with apple sauce or sour cream

Recipe makes 24 pancakes. All values are per serving (2 pancakes). **Calories: 301**, Protein: 3g, Total Fat: 24g, Saturated Fat: 2g

1 Tbsp Applesauce adds 12 calories, 0g protein, 0g fat, 0g saturated fat

1 Tbsp Sour Cream adds 26 calories, 0g protein, 3g fat, 2g saturated fat

Desserts

Almond Candy Cookies

Contributed By: Kusum Naik

Total Time: 30 Minutes

Ingredients:

1 cup almonds (blended until finely chopped)

1 cup Carnation® powder milk

¾ cup sugar

¾ cup water

Directions:

Mix sugar with water and boil at medium-high temperature approximately 20 minutes

Place a drop of vanilla extract in the syrup

Check the syrup (sugar/water) consistency by placing on a spoon. If it stays on the spoon, it is the correct consistency; if it runs off, cook longer

Add syrup to the almond and carnation powder mixture – mix immediately with two spoons

Continue to add syrup and mix until dough-like consistency.

Turn off the stove

Let it cool a bit so you can handle

Place warm water on hands and then make small handfuls of almond candy cookies and place on wax paper

Store this in the refrigerator and enjoy!

Recipe makes 20 cookies. All values are per cookie. **Calories: 50**, Protein: 2g, Total Fat: 0g, Saturated Fat: 0g

Apple Cobbler Pie

Contributed By: Carol Day

Total Time: 1 Hour and 10 Minutes

Ingredients for Filling and Pie Crust:

1 9″ prepared pie crust

6 large or 9 small McIntosh apples peeled and sliced

2 cup sour cream

1 cup sugar

2 eggs

½ tsp salt

2 Tbsp vanilla

½ cup flour

Ingredients for Topping:

½ cup brown sugar

½ cup sugar

½ cup flour

1 Tbsp cinnamon

1 cup chopped walnuts

½up butter

Directions:

Mix filling and put in 10 inch prepared pie shell

Bake 450° F for 10 minutes

Then reduce oven temperature to 350° F and bake for 35-40 minutes

Meanwhile, blend all the topping ingredients

When the baking is done, place the topping on top of the pie

Bake for 15 minutes at 350° F

Serve with vanilla ice cream….tastes good warm

Recipe makes 8 servings. All values are per serving. **Calories: 732**, Protein: 9g, Total Fat: 42g, Saturated Fat: 17g

½ cup premium **vanilla ice cream adds 184 calories**, 3g protein, 12g Total fat, 8g Saturated fat

Baked Custard

Contributed By: Evelyn Scher

Total Time: 55 Minutes

Ingredients:

3 eggs

¼ cup sugar

¼ teaspoon salt

2 cups milk, scalded

½ teaspoon vanilla

Directions:

Start oven at moderate (325° F) temperature

Combine eggs, sugar and salt

Add milk and vanilla slowly

Pour into 6 (5 ounce) custard cups

Set cups in shallow pan containing about 1 inch hot water

Bake 40 to 45 minutes or until knife inserted in center of cup comes out clean

Serve warm or chilled

Recipe makes 6 servings. All values are per serving. **Calories: 117**, Protein: 6g, Total Fat: 5g, Saturated Fat: 2g

Banana Bread with Chocolate Chips

Contributed By: Rhonda Levy

Total Time: 1 Hour and 20 Minutes

Ingredients:

½ cup butter

2 eggs

1 tsp baking soda

1 cup mashed bananas (3, very ripe)

1 cup sugar

2 cups flour

½ tsp cinnamon

½ tsp salt

½ cup chocolate chips

Directions:

Cream butter and sugar thoroughly

Add egg, beating until blended

Sift together dry ingredients and add to mixture

Blend in bananas and chocolate chips

Pour mixture into a greased 9 X 5 loaf pan and bake in a 350° F oven for 1 hour

Cool slightly before removing from pan

Recipe makes 8 servings. All values are per serving. **Calories: 358**, Protein:5g, Total Fat: 14g, Saturated Fat: 8g

Black Bottom Cupcakes

Contributed By: Barbara Reiff

Total Time: 40 Minutes

Ingredients:

¼ cup cocoa

1½ cup flour

1/3 cup vegetable oil

1 tsp baking soda

1 tsp vanilla

1 cup water

1 cup sugar

Ingredients for Filling:

1 8 oz package of cream cheese

1/3 cup of Sugar

1 Egg

6 oz mini chocolate chips

Directions:

Preheat oven to 350° F

In a large bowl, combine cocoa, flour, oil, baking soda, vanilla, water, and sugar until smooth

In a smaller bowl, combine cream cheese, sugar and egg until smooth.

Stir in chocolate chips

Line a 12 cup cupcake pan with paper liners. Pour equal amounts of chocolate mixture in each cup. Top with equal amounts of cream cheese mixture.

Bake for 20-25 minutes

Recipe makes 12 cupcakes. All values are per cupcake. **Calories: 328,** Protein: 4g, Total Fat: 17g, Saturated Fat: 8g

Carrot Cake

Contributed By: Patti Gelman

Total Time: 90 Minutes

Ingredients for Carrot Cake:

2 cup all-purpose flour

2 tsp baking powder

1 ½ tsp baking soda

1 tsp salt

2 tsp ground cinnamon

1 ¾ cup granulated sugar

1 ½ cup vegetable oil

4 eggs

2 cup grated carrots

½ cup walnuts (optional)

1 cup crushed and drained pineapple (reserve juice for icing)

Directions:

Preheat oven to 350° F. Grease and flour two 9″ round cake pans (I sometimes use a tube pan)

In a large bowl, stir together flour, baking powder, baking soda, salt and cinnamon

In another large bowl, mix sugar and oil; beat in eggs with an electric mixer. Stir in carrots, nuts (optional) and pineapple. Stir in flour mixture. Pour into prepared pans.

Ingredients for Cream Cheese Icing:

1 lb cream cheese

½ cup butter, softened

2 tsp vanilla extract

2 ½ cups confectioner's sugar

3 Tbsp pineapple juice

Directions:

In a large bowl, cream together butter and cream cheese with an electric mixer

Add vanilla and mix

Add pineapple juice and mix well (I sometimes return the icing to the fridge to firm it up a bit before spreading on the cake if it seems runny and keep the cake in the fridge after it is finished)

Bake for 45 minutes at 350° F, or until a cake tester inserted in center comes out clean

Remove pans to wire rack to cool 15 minutes before removing cake from pans

Finish cooling; then ice

Recipe makes 12 Servings. All values are per serving. **Calories: 791**, Protein: 8g, Total Fat: 53 g, Saturated Fat: 18 g

Chocolate Brownies

Contributed By: Rhonda Levy

Total Time: 55 Minutes

Ingredients:

10 oz package of chocolate chips

1 cup sugar

1/3 cup butter

2 Tbsp water

2 large eggs

1 tsp vanilla extract

3/4 cup flour

1/2 tsp salt

Colored sprinkles to match the season, holiday, etc

8 inch square baking pan

Directions:

Preheat oven to 325° F

Heat 1 cup chocolate chips, sugar, butter and water over low heat, stirring constantly until melted

Pour mixture into a bowl and add eggs, one at a time. Add vanilla, then flour and salt

Mix well

Add the rest of the chocolate chips

Pour into greased 8 x 8 inch pan

Sprinkle the sprinkles on top

Bake for 35 minutes

Cut into 1″ squares

Recipe makes 8 servings. **Calories: 400**, Protein: 3g Total Fat: 18g, Saturated Fat: 13g

Chocolate Chip Cheesecake

Contributed By: Carol Day

Total Time: 1 hour 15 minutes

Ingredients for Crust:

¾ cup ground walnuts

¾ cup graham crackers

3 Tbsp melted butter

Directions for Crust:

Mix crust ingredients together and press in the bottom of a 9 inch spring form pan

Ingredients for Filling:

1 can (14-oz) Eagle brand sweetened condensed milk (not evaporated milk)

3 eggs

2 tsp vanilla extract

1 cup mini chocolate chips

1 tsp flour

Directions for Filling:

Preheat oven to 300° F

In large mixing bowl, beat cheese until fluffy

Add Eagle® Brand Condensed Milk and beat until smooth

Add eggs and vanilla: mix well

In small bowl, toss together 1/2 cup chips with flour to coat; stir into cheese mixture

Pour mixture into prepared pan

Sprinkle remaining chips evenly over the top

Bake 1 hour or until cake springs back when lightly touched

Cool at room temperature and chill

Remove side of pan. Garnish as desired. Refrigerate leftovers

Recipe makes 8 servings. All values are per serving. **Calories: 373,** Protein: 6g, Total Fat: 16g, Saturated Fat: 8g

Date Almond Delight

Contributed By: Kusum Naik

Total Time: 45 Minutes

Ingredients:

20 dates (cut into small pieces)

3 Tbsp butter

1 cup almonds (finely chopped)

1 can sweet condensed milk

Directions:

Place cut up dates into pan with 3 Tbsp butter

Cook on low temperature about 5 minutes until butter is melted and dates soften

Add chopped nuts

Add 1 can sweet condensed milk

Cook until dough like consistency

Turn off stove

Remove dough and place on wax paper positioned in a log

Allow the dough to cool down and harden a bit

Slice into bite size delights

Recipe makes 24 Delights. All values are per serving. **Calories: 93**, Protein: 1g, Total Fat: 4g, Saturated Fat: 1g

Devil Dog Recipe

Contributed By: Barbara Reiff

Total Time: 35 Minutes

Ingredients for cake:

2 cup Flour

1 cup Sugar

½ cup unsweetened cocoa

1 tsp baking soda

½ tsp baking powder

½ tsp salt

½ cup sour milk (1½ tsp lemon juice in 1 cup of milk. Let stand 5 minutes)

½ cup water

½ cup butter

1 egg

1 egg yolk

Ingredients for filling:

½ cup butter

2 tsp vanilla

2 Tbsp flour

3 Tbsp milk

1 Tbsp sugar

2 ½ cup powdered sugar

Directions for cake:

Preheat oven to 400° F

Combine sugar, flour, cocoa, soda, powder and salt

Add milk, water and butter. Beat until combined. Beat 2 more minutes on medium

Add eggs, beat 2 more minutes

Drop by teaspoon on ungreased cookie sheet and bake for 5 minutes

Directions for filling:

Mix butter, flour and vanilla. Beat for 30 seconds

Add ½ the powdered sugar, then the milk, then remainder of powdered sugar

Spread filling between 2 cakes to form Devil Dogs

Recipe makes 18 servings. All values are per serving. **Calories: 267,** Protein: 3g, Total Fat: 12g, Saturated Fat: 7g

Fruit Cobbler

Contributed By: Jan Zauzmer

Total Time: 1 Hour and 15 Minutes

Ingredients:

1 cup flour

1 cup sugar

¼ tsp salt

2 tsp baking powder

¾ cup milk

½ cup butter

2 cans fruit filling in fruit of your choice

Carton vanilla ice cream

Directions:

Mix flour, sugar, salt, and baking powder

Add milk and melted butter and beat until smooth

Pour into 2-qt baking shallow dish greased with margarine

Add fruit

Bake at 350° F for about an hour until batter magically rises to top to cover fruit and browns

Serve warm with vanilla ice cream for an easy dessert

Recipe makes 8 servings. All values are per serving. **Calories: 442**, Protein: 3g, Total Fat: 16g, Saturated Fat: 8g

½ cup premium vanilla **ice cream adds 184 calories**, 3g protein, 12g total fat, 8g saturated fat

Mississippi Mud or Dirt Pie

Contributed By: Carol Day

Total Time: 1 Hour

Ingredients:

1 ½ sticks of butter or margarine

1 ½ cup of flour

2 cups or more chopped nuts

8 oz cream cheese

1 large container of Cool Whip®

1 cup confectionary sugar

2 boxes instant chocolate pudding

3 ½ cups milk

Gummy worms for decoration

Directions First layer:

1 ½ stick of butter/margarine

1 ½ cups of flour

1 ½ cups chopped nuts

Mix butter and flour and nuts

Press into 9 X 13 inch pan

Bake 25-30 minutes @ 350° F

Cool and then refrigerate until cool

Directions Second layer:

8 ounces of cream cheese

1 cup cool whip

1 cup confectionary sugar

Mix cream cheese and sugar: add cool whip and spread over first layer

Directions Third layer:

2 boxes of instant chocolate pudding using 3½ cups of milk

Mix according to the box and pour over second layer

Cool

Directions Fourth layer:

Cover with the cool whip and nuts

Kids like gummy worms on top to decorate the dirt

Recipe makes 12 servings. All values are per serving. **Calories: 626**, Protein: 9g, Total Fat: 41g, Saturated Fat: 16g

Pumpkin Tiramisu

Contributed By: Debbie Kaufman

Total Time: 40 Minutes plus overnight refrigeration

Start One Day Ahead for this recipe

Ingredients:

1 ½ cups chilled whipping cream

¾ cup sugar

8 oz cream cheese

15 oz can pure pumpkin

¾ tsp pumpkin pie spice (or ¼ tsp each cinnamon, cloves, and nutmeg)

2 3 oz packages halved ladyfingers

2 oz crushed amaretti cookies

Directions:

Beat 1½ cups chilled whipping cream and ¾ cup sugar until peaks form.

Add one 8 oz container mascarpone cheese, one 15 ounce can pure pumpkin and ¾ teaspoon pumpkin pie spice (or substitute as outlined above). Beat until filling is smooth.

Line bottom of 9 inch diameter spring form pan with one 3 ounce package halved ladyfingers, overlapping and crowding to fit

Sprinkle with 2 Tbsp rum (optional).

Spread half of filling over ladyfingers

Repeat with one 3 oz package halved ladyfingers, 2 Tbsp rum (optional) and remaining filling. Smooth

Wrap tightly in plastic, then foil

Chill overnight

To unmold, run knife around inside edge of pan. Release pan sides and sprinkle with 2 ounces crushed Amaretti cookies

Recipe makes 8 servings. All values are per serving. **Calories: 321**, Protein: 4g, Total Fat: 19g, Saturated Fat: 11g

Watermelon Nut Delight

Contributed By: Kusum Naik

Total Time: 2 hours

Ingredients:

1 ⅓cup Carnation® Powder Milk

Mini chocolate sprinkle

1 cup ground (powder) almonds (raw without salt)

Vanilla extract (optional)

1 cup ground (powder) pistachios (raw without salt)

Rose Extract (optional)

2 cup ground (powder) cashews (raw without salt)

1 ⅓cup cup sugar

Red food coloring

1 ⅓ cup water

Green food coloring

¼ cup Chocolate sprinkles

Directions:

Mix ⅓ cup milk powder with almond powder in a bowl.

Mix ⅓ milk powder with pistachio powder in a bowl

Mix ⅔ milk powder with cashew powder in a bowl.

For Almond

Mix ⅓ cup sugar with ⅓ cup of water and boil at medium-high temperature approximately 8 minutes to make syrup

Place few drops of red food coloring in the syrup and rose extract (optional)

Check the syrup (sugar/water) consistency by placing on a spoon. (if it does not spread on the spoon, it is the correct consistency; if it runs off, cook longer)

Add almond mixture to the syrup

Turn off the heat and mix until dough-like consistency

Set aside to cool

For Pistachio

Mix ⅓ cup sugar with ⅓ cup of water and boil at medium-high temperature approximately 8 minutes to make syrup

Place few drops of green food coloring in the syrup

Check the syrup (sugar/water) consistency by placing on a spoon (if it does not spread on the spoon, it is the correct consistency; if it runs off, cook longer

Add cashew mixture to the syrup

Turn off the heat and mix until dough-like consistency

Set aside to cool

For Cashew

Mix ⅔ cup sugar with ⅔ cup of water and boil at medium-high temperature approximately 10 min to make syrup

Place a few drops of vanilla extract (optional)

Check the syrup (sugar/water) consistency by placing on a spoon. If it does not spread on the spoon, it is the correct consistency; if it runs off, cook longer

Add cashew mixture to the syrup. Turn off the heat and mix until dough-like consistency

Set aside to cool

Directions for presentation:

Let it cool a bit so you can handle

Add chocolate sprinkles in the almond nut mix (red color)

Knead all three different kinds of dough separately

Create 4 balls of each color mix (Red (almond), Green (Pistachio) and natural (cashew)

To create a watermelon look, you will be sculpting each color of balled dough over the next color as outlined below:

Pick up one of the red almond nut mix balls

Roll each of the cashew dough ball (natural color) between saran wrap with roller pin and cover it over each red ball (you will need to judge how much you want to roll to be able to cover the red/white ball)

Roll each of the pistachio dough balls (green color) between saran wrap with roller pin and cover it over the natural color ball (you will need to judge how much you want to roll to be able to cover the red/white ball)

Refrigerate

Cut in slices

Yield approx. 40 pieces (10 pieces per ball)

Recipe makes 40 pieces. All values are per piece. **Calories: 154** , Protein: 5g, Total Fat: 16g , Saturated Fat: 2g

12 East Cheesecake

Contributed By: David Reiff

Total Time: 1 Hour and 15 Minutes plus overnight refrigeration if desired

Ingredients for Crust:

1/8 pound melted butter (1/2 stick)

1 ½ cups graham cracker crumbs

¼ cup sugar

Ingredients for Cheesecake:

2 8 oz packages of cream cheese

½ cup sugar

3 eggs

¾ tsp vanilla

Ingredients for Topping (optional):

1 pint sour cream

1 tsp vanilla

¼ cup sugar

Optional strawberries or blueberries

Directions to prepare Crust:

Mix ingredients

Pack down to form crust in pan or cheesecake form

Bake at 325° F for 5 minutes

Cool in refrigerator for 20 minutes

Directions to prepare Cheesecake:

Mix together by hand, then beat with mixer 7 minutes

Pour mixture over crust, then bake at 375° F for 20-30 minutes

Remove from oven and let cool for 10 minutes

Refrigerate 12 hours (unless topping, then see next page)

To prepare Topping (optional):

Mix topping ingredients

Place on top of cheesecake that's been cooled for 10 minutes

Bake at 475° F for 5 minutes

Refrigerate 12 hours

Recipe makes 8 Servings. All values are per serving. **Calories: 573**, Protein: 10g, Total Fat: 40g, Saturated Fat: 24g

Chapter 7 - Calorie Rich Drinks

What You Should Know about Drinks, Shakes and Other Liquid-based Foods!

While liquid-based nutrition supplements can be and have been a godsend for many people who are unable to take in adequate calories and nutrition from solid foods, there are some things you should know about how fluids and liquids affect appetite. First, many people prefer to consume their calories and nutrition in this form when they are feeling nauseous or disinterested in food. This is likely because it seems **easier** to drink than eat calories during such times. However, drinks and liquid based foods can make you feel fuller than you really might be because they take up more space and volume in your stomach than other foods. For example, think about how different your stomach would feel after you ate a handful of nuts or chips compared to after drinking a large milkshake or a gallon of water. Many people do not realize that any liquid-based foods, even soup, can have this "filling" effect. So be careful about not drinking too much or consuming too many liquid-based foods as they could actually interfere further with your appetite for solid foods. Another example of this is little children who drink juice all day long and parents claim they are not hungry or they just do not eat. If the juice intake is decreased, their appetite for solid foods almost always improves.

At times people do not have a choice and must rely solely on liquid nutrition. If this is the case, it is especially important that you try to get the most "bang-for-your-buck" with everything you do drink. That is, try to ensure that it is as calorie and nutrient dense as possible. Instead of just drinking plain juice or water, try to drink juices fortified with additional vitamins and minerals and/or added protein. Consider making your own shakes with calorie and nutrient dense ingredients (recipes provided in this section). It is also important to try to be creative and get as much flavor variety as possible to prevent "taste fatigue" – a common condition that occurs when people eat or drink the same food over and over again, particularly when eating or drinking the food is not by choice, but by necessity. We hope you enjoy some of the delicious and nutritious "liquid" food choices we have provided in the following pages.

ICE CREAM OR COLD ENERGY DRINKS

For all drinks, use blender to mix to desired consistency

Apple Pie A La Mode

½ cup milk

ADD

1 cup apple pie filling

1 cup vanilla ice cream

Dash of cinnamon

Calories: 289 calories

Black and White Milk Shake

½ cup vanilla ice cream

¾ cup milk

ADD

3 Tbsp chocolate sauce

1 tsp vanilla extract

Calories: 444

Boost® Apricot Peach Smoothie

½ cup (½ bottle) BOOST® Vanilla

ADD

2/3 cup apricot nectar

½ cup peaches, sliced

Ice

Calories: 250

Boost® Blueberry Blast

1-8 fl oz bottle BOOST® Vanilla

ADD

2 tsp creamy peanut butter

2 tsp grape jelly

½ cup vanilla or peanut butter swirl ice cream

Calories: 450

Boost® Chocolate Coconut Delight

½ cup (1/2 bottle) BOOST® Vanilla

ADD

½ cup coconut milk, chilled

1/8 tsp almond extract

½ cup chocolate ice cream

Calories: 480

Boost® Creamy Pina Colada

8 fl oz bottle BOOST® Vanilla

ADD

2 tsp cream of coconut

1/8 tsp coconut extract

½ cup crushed pineapple, drained

½ cup chopped ice

Calories: 320

Boost® Fuzzy Navel

8 fl oz bottle BOOST® Vanilla

ADD

½ cup sliced frozen peaches

2 Tbsp frozen orange juice concentrate

Calories: 280

Boost® Guava Banana

½ cup (1/2 bottle) BOOST® Vanilla

ADD

2/3 cup guava nectar

½ ripe banana, frozen banana

Ice

Calories: 270

Boost® Mango Tango

8 fl oz bottle BOOST® Vanilla or Strawberry

ADD

½ cup (1/2 bottle) BOOST Vanilla

½ cup mango or guava nectar, chilled

¾ cup mango, diced

Ice

Calories: 270

Boost® Nutty Butter Banana Shake

8 fl oz bottle BOOST® Vanilla

ADD

1 tsp creamy peanut butter

1 banana, sliced and frozen

½ cup vanilla or peanut butter swirl ice cream

Calories: 510

Boost® PB & J Milkshake

8 fl oz bottle BOOST® Vanilla

ADD

2 tsp creamy peanut butter

1 tsp grape jelly

½ cup vanilla or peanut butter swirl ice cream

Calories: 470

Boost® Peach Perfection

8 fl oz bottle BOOST® Vanilla

ADD

¾ cup peaches (in heavy syrup), sliced

½ cup vanilla ice cream

Calories: 420

Boost® Pumpkin Nog

8 oz bottle BOOST® Vanilla

ADD

½ cup solid pack pumpkin

1 Tbsp honey

½ tsp cinnamon

1 cup vanilla ice cream

Rum, optional

Calories: 600

Boost® Strawberry Banana

8 fl oz bottle BOOST® Vanilla or Strawberry

ADD

1 banana, sliced

½ cup strawberries, sliced

½ cup vanilla ice cream or low fat frozen yogurt

Calories: 500

Chocolate Milk Shake

½ cup Chocolate Ice Cream

¾ cup milk

2 Tbsp chocolate syrup

ADD

Blend to yield 1 milk shake

Calories: 398

Chocolate-Peanut Butter Shake

1 packet Carnation® Breakfast Essentials™ powder

ADD

½ cup heavy whipping cream

3 Tbsp creamy peanut butter

3 Tbsp chocolate syrup

1 ½ cup chocolate ice cream

Calories: 914

Coco Coco Shake

2 Tbsp Cream of Coconut

ADD

1 Tbsp chocolate fudge sauce

½ cup Premium Vanilla Ice Cream

1 tsp vanilla or almond extract

¾ cup whole milk

Calories: 496

Creamsicle

½ cup Vanilla Ice Cream

ADD

¾ cup milk

½ tsp vanilla

¼ cup orange sherbet

Calories: 347

Great Grape Slush

½ cup whole milk

ADD

2 grape juice bars

2 tsp corn syrup

1 Tbsp corn oil

Calories: 316

High Calorie Carnation® Shake

½ cup half & half

ADD

¾ cup ice cream

1 packet Carnation® Breakfast Essentials™ powder

3 Tbsp peanut butter

Calories: 860

Ice Coffee

½ cup Coffee Ice Cream

ADD

¾ cup milk

2 tsp coffee syrup

Calories: 392

Orange Sherbet Shake

1 packet Vanilla Carnation® Breakfast Essentials™ powder

ADD

¾ cup orange sherbet

½ cup whole milk

2 tsp corn syrup

2 tbsp corn oil

Calories: 643

Peaches & Cream

1 cup milk

ADD

1 cup canned peaches

1 cup rich vanilla ice cream

¼ tsp salt

¼ tsp vanilla

Calories: 359

Raspberry

½ cup Vanilla Ice Cream

ADD

¾ cup milk

½ tsp vanilla

1/8 cup Melba sauce

Calories: 399

Root Beer Float

½ cup full-fat ice cream

ADD

6 oz root beer

Place ice cream in mug

Pour root beer over ice cream

Calories: 260

Scandi Appleberry Punch

¾ cup strawberry SCANDISHAKE®

ADD

4 ounces apple juice

4 ounces cranberry juice

Calories: 460 calories

Scandi Banana Shake

½ cup vanilla SCANDISHAKE®

ADD

½ cup whole milk

½ small ripe banana and ½ tsp banana flavoring

Calories: 572 calories

½ cup Premium vanilla ice cream

2 T evaporated whole milk

Scandi Coconut Cider

½ cup vanilla SCANDISHAKE®

ADD

6 ounces apple cider

¼ C canned coconut milk

1 teaspoon vanilla

Dash cinnamon

Calories: 428 calories

Scandi Coconut Cream Pie

¼ cup vanilla SCANDISHAKE®

ADD

½ cup whole milk

2 T evaporated whole milk

¼ cup coconut milk

Top with 2 teaspoons grated coconut

2 ½ tsp vanilla extract

½ cup premium vanilla ice cream

Calories: 566

Scandi Cranorange Shake

¾ cup vanilla SCANDISHAKE®

ADD

3 oz orange juice

5 oz cranberry juice

Calories: 461 calories

Scandi Eggnog

1/4 cup vanilla SCANDISHAKE®

ADD

3/4 cup purchased eggnog drink

¼ cup half and half

¼ tsp vanilla extract

Dash cinnamon and nutmeg for garnish

Calories: 445

Scandi Fruit Spritzer

½ cup strawberry SCANDISHAKE®

¼ cup whole milk

4 ice cubes made from ginger ale

Mix Ginger ice cubes, milk and SCANDISHAKE® in a blender

ADD

¼ cup frozen raspberries

¼ cup frozen mango

½ small ripe banana (add fruit into blender)

ADD

½ cup ginger ale and stir gently so drink is fizzy

Calories: 432

Scandi Lemon Drop

½ cup vanilla SCANDISHAKE®

ADD

¼ cup buttermilk

½ cup premium vanilla ice cream

½ cup lemonade

2 ounces frozen lemonade concentrate

Calories: 664 calories

Scandi Orange Creamsickle

½ cup vanilla SCANDISHAKE®

ADD

½ cup premium vanilla ice cream

2 T evaporated whole milk

½ cup orange juice

Calories: 502

Scandi Orange Julius

¼ cup vanilla SCANDISHAKE®

ADD

½ cup half and half

2 T sweetened lime juice

¼ cup orange juice

½ cup orange sherbet

Calories: 462

Scandi Peach Pie

½ cup vanilla SCANDISHAKE®

ADD

¼ cup whole milk

¼ cup frozen peaches

2 ½ tsp vanilla extract

½ cup premium Caramel ice cream

½ cup peach nectar

Top with crushed graham crackers (not made with honey)

Calories: 648

Scandi Raspberry Twist

¼ cup vanilla SCANDISHAKE®

½ cup half and half

2 ounces cranberry juice

ADD

2 T sweetened lime juice

½ cup raspberry sherbet

¼ cup frozen raspberries in syrup

Calories: 582 calories

Scandi Strawberry Fields

¼ cup strawberry SCANDISHAKE®

ADD

½ cup strawberry premium ice cream

½ cup whole milk

¼ cup fresh or frozen strawberries

¼ cup coconut milk

Calories: 583

Scandi Strawberry Fountain Shake

½ cup vanilla SCANDISHAKE®

ADD

½ cup whole milk

½ cup premium strawberry ice cream

2 T strawberry syrup

2 T evaporated whole milk

Calories: 695

Strawberry Crush

2 Tbsp honey

ADD

2 cups frozen strawberries

½ cup crushed pineapple

½ cup water

½ medium banana

6 Tbsp sugar

¼ cup lemon juice

Calories: 324

Tropical Fruit Delight

Recipe makes 4 servings

1 ½ oz Cream of Coconut

ADD

10 oz frozen strawberries

32 oz can pineapple juice

4 lemon wedges

Calories: 235

Blend Berries and pineapple juice on low speed.

Garnish with lemon

Vanilla Milk Shake

½ cup full fat ice cream

¾ cup whole milk

ADD

¾ tsp vanilla extract

Blend to yield 1 milk shake

Calories: 294

(Calories are based on full fat premium ice cream)

HOT DRINKS

Caution: blend ingredients together before heating in microwave to avoid burns

Café Con Leche

Mix:

4 oz brewed coffee

2 oz evaporated milk

1 tsp canola oil

Calories: 132

Café Mocha

4 oz brewed coffee

2 oz evaporated milk

1 tsp canola oil

2 tsp chocolate syrup

Calories: 165

Cranberry Spiced Cider

6 oz apple cider (pasteurized)

2 Tbsp jellied cranberry sauce

1 tsp canola oil

¼ tsp lemon zest

Calories: 165

Dulche de Leche

6 oz whole milk

3 Tbsp caramel sauce

1 tsp canola oil

1 tsp vanilla

Calories: 340

Emily's Banana Cream Pie

1 Tbsp mashed bananas

6 oz whole milk

2 oz evaporated milk

1tsp vanilla

2 Nilla wafers crushed for the top

Calories: 253

Heavenly Hot Chocolate

3 oz milk chocolate (melted)

ADD

1 tsp butter (melted)

¼ tsp vanilla

1 cup half & half

Calories: 802

Hot Apple Cider

6 oz cider (pasteurized)

2 Tbsp apple butter or apple puree

2 tsp canola oil

Dash of cinnamon

Calories: 364

Hot Vanilla Not Chocolate

6 oz whole milk

2 oz evaporated milk

1 tsp butter (melted)

1 tsp vanilla

Calories: 230

Oreos® and Coconut Cream

6 oz whole milk

2 oz coconut milk

1 Oreo® cookie crushed

1 Tbsp shredded coconut

Calories: 318

Pumpkin Pie a La Talia

1 oz pumpkin puree

4 oz whole milk

1 oz evaporated milk

2 tsp maple syrup

Once heated, add ice cream prior to serving

1 scoop (1/2 cup) vanilla, caramel or pumpkin ice cream

Pumpkin Spice mix to taste

Calories: 351

©/™ Nestle', reprinted with permission.

ScandiShake® trademark is owned by Aptalis Pharma US, Inc. Trademarks are reserved to their respective owners. Scandishake can be ordered at www.aptalispharma.com.

Nutrition Data for all contributed recipes provided by Axxya Systems-Nutritionist Pro ™ www.axxya.com using version 8.0 Diet Analysis + version.

Logo Design by Bailey Brand Consulting

Cover Design by Jason Alexander of Expert Subjects, LLC

HOW TO CONTACT US:

For additional information or to share stories:

Email:	cravingcaloriesllc@gmail.com
Website:	www.cravingcalories.com
Facebook:	www.facebook.com/cravingcaloriescookbook
Blog:	www.cravingcalories.wordpress.com
Linkedin:	www.linkedin.com/company/craving-calories-llc
Twitter:	www.twitter.com/cravingcalories

To order an e-book or additional print copies of this book, visit: www.cravingcalories.com

Contact us to share your successes, thoughts and recipe ideas.

We hope that you found this book informative and helpful. We would love to hear from you.

Debbie *LaurieAnn* *Melanie*

40428654R00116

Made in the USA
Lexington, KY
05 April 2015